What People Are Saying About Dr. Henry W. Wright and *Exposing the Spiritual Roots of Disease...*

In *Exposing the Spiritual Roots of Disease*, Dr. Henry Wright destroys the lie that we are helpless victims of diseases that afflict us randomly, and empowers us to take responsibility for our health in partnership with the Holy Spirit. As a general medical practitioner, I fully endorse the notion that, as triune beings, we can only truly be healthy when we are whole in spirit, soul, and body. This book is long overdue and is essential reading for any Christian struggling with sickness and for those who seek to minister to them.

—Dr. Rebecca Williams, MA, MB ChB, DRCOG, DCH, DTM&H

Why are Christians experiencing the same disease rate as non-Christians? Why does prayer not heal everyone? Where does disease come from, and how can we live the life of freedom that God has planned for us? These are questions that Dr. Henry Wright addresses in *Exposing the Spiritual Roots of Disease*. When even the most trusted medical textbooks include "unknown etiology" (cause) for many diseases, where do we go for answers? In this book, Dr. Wright uses a solid scriptural base to reveal the roots of disease and give clear guidance on how we can be set free in spirit, soul, and body!

—Sheila Pitcock, LVN

I have followed Dr. Wright's ministry for three years and it has been life changing. With his second book, *Exposing the Spiritual Roots of Disease*, he answers questions that mankind has been searching for since the days of the ancient Egyptians. We always want to get to the bottom of things— "Get to the root," we say—but no one until now has done that when it comes to sickness and disease. The medical field does not understand the connection between spirit, soul, and body; consequently, they are of little help. But now we have the answers! This complex subject is made simple by Dr. Wright's easy-to-read book, which gives people hope where there has not been hope before! A must-read!

—Rev. Dr. S. R. Watkins, PhD, New Start Ministries

In *Exposing the Spiritual Roots of Disease*, Dr. Henry Wright pulls back the curtain and explains—with science and Scripture—why we get sick. Then, he gives us real tools from Scripture to prevent us from becoming sick in the first place. Thousands of people have gotten their lives back as a result of this teaching—and now you can too. Read this book and apply what you read. Then, prepare to be amazed by the results.

—Robert McFarland, President, Transformational Impact LLC;
Blogger-in-Chief, RobertMcFarland.net;
best-selling author, *Dear Boss: What Your Employees Wish You Knew* and
Dear Employee: What Your Boss Wishes You Knew

Dr. Henry Wright has done research over a long period of time and gives answers to questions about diseases and their spiritual roots. In my profession as a therapist for people who are addicted and people with psychiatric problems, I need answers as to how to be able to help them—not just managing the disease, but really giving solutions. I am deeply grateful for this revelation.

—Frans Izeboud, Addictions Therapist
BA in Social Work, MA Family Therapist, Psychiatric Social Coach

Here's your wake-up call, church! Have you ever wondered why God's people are as sick as the world and dying of the same diseases as unbelievers? In *Exposing the Spiritual Roots of Disease*, Dr. Henry Wright has sounded the alarm for believers to shift their focus from healing to disease prevention! It is truly God's heart for us that we would never need healing. The Scriptures and insights that Dr. Wright shares in this work are a compilation of thirty-plus years of biblical study and personal observation while caring for the flock as a pastor. *Exposing the Spiritual Roots of Disease* is just what the doctor ordered to adjust our spiritual misalignments and restore proper body alignment under the Head, which is Christ Jesus, so we can be healed, remain whole, and be in health.

—Pastor Travis Wortham, DC, BS

In his new book, *Exposing the Spiritual Roots of Disease*, Dr. Henry Wright states, "You should be a thriver! While the world might be struggling in disease and hopelessness, you should be a happy, well-balanced, and enthusiastic son or daughter of God." To accomplish this, you must realize that we are engaged in a spiritual war with Satan that requires the use of knowledge in order to defeat the enemy. This book will change the way you think and act because it reveals a journey of healing that occurs from the inside out—understanding the spiritual roots of many diseases, utilizing the knowledge of biblical truth, and relying on God's Word as the lamp for your journey in life. Dr. Wright lays out this journey in a logical, pragmatic manner, reinforced with Scripture, real-life examples, and Christian solutions. Regardless of where you are in your journey, or the knowledge that you currently possess, this is a must-read book!

—Dr. Michael Costello, Associate Professor,
School of Applied Engineering and Technology College of Engineering,
Southern Illinois University Carbondale

DR. HENRY W. WRIGHT

BEST-SELLING AUTHOR OF *A MORE EXCELLENT WAY*

REVISED AND EXPANDED EDITION

EXPOSING THE SPIRITUAL ROOTS OF DISEASE

POWERFUL ANSWERS TO YOUR QUESTIONS ABOUT HEALING AND DISEASE PREVENTION

WHITAKER
HOUSE

All Scripture quotations are taken from the King James Version of the Holy Bible.

The forms Lord and God (in small capital letters) in Bible quotations represent the Hebrew name for God *Yahweh* (Jehovah), while *Lord* and *God* normally represent the name *Adonai*.

Exposing the Spiritual Roots of Disease:
Powerful Answers to Your Questions About Healing and Disease Prevention
Second Edition: Revised and Expanded

Be in Health®, LLC
4178 Crest Highway, Thomaston, GA 30286
www.beinhealth.com
info@beinhealth.com

ISBN: 979-8-88769-035-3
eBook ISBN: 978-1-64123-334-7
Printed in the United States of America
© 2019, 2023 by Be in Health®, LLC. All rights reserved.

Whitaker House
1030 Hunt Valley Circle
New Kensington, PA 15068
www.whitakerhouse.com

Library of Congress Control Number: 2023934638

1 2 3 4 5 6 7 8 9 10 11 ᴧ 30 29 28 27 26 25 24 23

CONTENTS

DISCLAIMER

We do not seek to be in conflict with any medical or psychiatric practices, or any church or its religious doctrines, beliefs, or practices. We are not part of medicine or psychology; we are working to make them more effective, believing that many human problems are fundamentally spiritual, with associated physiological and psychological manifestations. This information is intended for your general knowledge only, to give insight into disease, its problems, and possible solutions. It is not a substitute for medical advice or treatment for specific medical conditions or disorders. We do not diagnose or treat disease.

You should seek prompt medical care for any specific health issues. Treatment modalities around your specific health issues are between you and your physician. We are not responsible for a person's disease or their healing. We are administering the Scriptures and what they say about this subject, along with what the medical and scientific communities have observed in line with this insight. There is no guarantee any person will be healed or any disease prevented. The fruits of this teaching will come forth out of the application of the principles and the relationship between each person and God. Be in Health˚ is patterned after 2 Corinthians 5:18–20, 1 Corinthians 12, Ephesians 4, and Mark 16:15–20.

FOREWORD

My husband, Dr. Henry W. Wright, was a brilliant man with a hunger for learning and an even stronger desire to serve God with all of his heart. He met the challenges of life with compassion, tough love, and his unique humor. It would be impossible to measure the impact he had on the lives of the people around him. His heart was to lead others to wholeness and peace in the love of God. He did his best to represent God's love in all that he did.

During his early years as a pastor, Henry's prayer was for answers to why physical healing from disease was not happening as often as it should in the church. That question, and God's answers, began his lifelong journey to exposing the spiritual roots of disease that were plaguing the body of Christ.

Henry spent decades researching biblical truths on what God said about healing, studying case histories of the people who came to the ministry for help, and learning about diseases and their effects on the human body from medical science. Together, we founded Be in Health and traveled throughout the United States and countries worldwide to teach biblical truths for overcoming diseases. The fantastic results were healing and restoration for tens of thousands of people across the globe. As the need for ministry increased, the For My Life Retreat was birthed. This impactful weeklong retreat on our church campus in Thomaston, Georgia, helps people understand the spiritual root causes of disease, apply the scriptural truths to their lives, and learn how to be set free!

Henry passed away in November 2019. Along with our family, church, and friends, I miss his presence every day. Shortly after Henry's passing, God spoke to my heart, "He's with Me, and he's good." Over five years ago, Henry and I, along with the Board of Elders, developed a plan to carry the biblical truths God had given him far into the future. Through Henry's relationship with the eldership and church body, we had a clear vision of how to move forward. Henry's vision was to establish generations of overcomers who would be restored—spirit, soul, and body—by God's Word and love.

Today, that is exactly what we are doing. The Be in Health team has expanded and continues to minister to thousands each month via our Thomaston, Georgia, campus, online seminars, mini-teachings, and conferences in cities across the country. The world is in great need of God's love and power to defeat the enemy and any diseases in their lives. We are pleased to present this revised and expanded edition of *Exposing the Spiritual Roots of Disease*. I hope the biblical insights Henry deposited in this book help lead you in your journey of healing and restoration.

—*Pastor Donna Wright*

FOREWORD

My introduction to Dr. Henry Wright's ministry came about in 2013 when my surgical technician gifted me a copy of Dr. Wright's book *A More Excellent Way*. Over the previous twenty years of practicing dermatology, I had pursued various theories and concepts concerning physical disease from psychology, nutrition, lifestyle change, and Eastern medicine. I found this approach quite commonly accepted by my patients. And yet, nothing enlightened my calling to work through the Word of the Lord Jesus Christ quite like Dr. Wright's insight.

His book explained that we all need the Father's love, which allows for transformation as we receive that love. The next step is to be aware of the potential spiritual roots of disease that, once recognized, can be removed. The process of removing the spiritual root is through Dr. Wright's "8 Rs to Freedom," which include recognition, taking responsibility, renouncing, repenting, removing, resisting, rejoicing, and restoring.

In the midst of weighing my present philosophies of medical practices against God's precepts, I was dealing with an unresolved inner conflict. Consequently, I developed a posterior vitreous detachment, which led to laser surgery in both eyes. Since my vocation was based on visual acuity, this condition had a major impact on the future of my career. I traveled to Thomaston, Georgia, to attend Dr. Henry Wright's For My Life Retreat.

This decision transformed both my physical well-being and my medical perspective forever. While at the conference, I discovered that my underlying spiritual issue was looking to man for answers instead of to God. Dr. Wright's preventative approach diverged from what I had experienced in the past. It incorporated the transformative power of God's Word and utilized the work of the Lord to not only manage disease but also to avoid it. His focus on disease prevention and cure rather than disease management resonated deeply with the direction I wanted to take for myself and my patients.

Since that conference, I have seen patients with a Holy Spirit-directed perspective. I utilize my medical training to diagnose and give a medically directed treatment plan, followed by a discussion of possible spiritual roots of disease that would be helpful to prevent recurrence, and with the hope to cure the disease. My goal now is to expose the underlying spiritual roots of my patients' diseases as often as I feel I am able. The patients who allow me to reach that next level of spiritual understanding of the disease and are made aware of the 8 Rs to Freedom have experienced miraculous changes.

I am eternally grateful to God for providing Dr. Henry Wright with this knowledge and insight to share with the world. I can say with full certainty that his teachings have transformed not only my life but the lives of my patients, as well.

I highly recommend Dr. Henry Wright's book *Exposing the Spiritual Roots of Disease* so that God may be glorified through each individual healed. I believe that Dr. Wright's insight into spiritual roots and pathways of disease, and his understanding of how to incorporate the 8 Rs to Freedom, will allow disease management to be minimized and disease cure to be maximized. I pray that this book will be read by physicians and other individuals who may normally feel hesitant toward receiving spiritual insight, so that patients can overcome their physical ailments based on the love and leading of Father God, Jesus the Word, and the Holy Spirit.

—*Barbara Schumann Bopp*, M.D.
Board Certified Dermatologist

INTRODUCTION: WHY ARE WE SICK?

Why are we sick?

In my journey to answer this question—to understand the root cause of disease—I have closely studied what God has said in His Word. During over thirty years of ministry, the most significant way I have impacted humans has been the result of reading my Bible, talking to Father God, and going out and helping people with the insights I have gleaned. It is really that simple. I firmly believe the crucial answers to humanity's diseases and problems have been laid out in the Bible for over thirty-five hundred years. Unfortunately, most people don't read the Bible to discover those answers.

I have also spent years studying the science of what God has created. The study of the human body is certainly essential in finding the root causes of disease. It is important to study what God has created, not just what He has said. Some people have accused me of being against science. Actually, I'm very indebted to science because it has enabled me to understand attributes and processes of the physical body that I would not have known otherwise. I may not always be in agreement with medicine's protocols for disease management, yet I am still grateful for what I have learned from scientific observation.

In my journey to understand disease, I have discovered that Western medicine concentrates on managing the symptoms of disease and disorders through drugs, therapies, and surgeries. With this method, it has developed advanced disease management, working to keep the disease under control. Then you have Eastern medicine, with its "natural," or alternative, treatments that attempt to manage the pathways that produce the symptoms of disease. But neither of these approaches represents true freedom from the disease itself. Neither answers the question of why we are sick.

The limitation of science is that scientists and medical professionals only address what they can see and measure. They are adept at accurately describing *how* we get sick. Their studies detail specific mechanisms of disease and biochemical malfunctions that disrupt our lives and our health.

In medical textbooks, a large number of diseases are listed with the name of the disease, the body parts affected, the diagnosis, the prognoses, and the protocols. At the end of these journal entries, a curious phrase is often inserted: "etiology unknown." Etiology refers to the root cause. They can see the disease, they can diagnose it, and they can track it—but they don't know or understand what triggers it. To find answers as to *why* our bodies' mechanisms malfunction, I look to the Bible. With God's leading and grace, we have spent decades tracking what causes or triggers disease. As a result of that knowledge, there have been literally thousands of people worldwide who have been freed of specific diseases and syndromes because they dealt with the root issues causing the manifestations.

I realize that the medical community is able to prove to you that living a stressful life is unhealthy. Their tests give us viable evidence of chemical imbalances due to living an anxiety-ridden life. These imbalances are causing problems throughout your body. Therefore, the purpose of most medications is to bring your body back to homeostasis or chemical balance. The medications may help you feel mostly normal, but they don't address *why* you were stressed out in the first place. As intelligent creatures, doesn't it make sense that we get down to the root cause that activated the pathways to disease in the first place? From there we can uproot it and be healed!

Now, what if I told you Father God could remove the problems in your life causing this stress so you do not need to be maintained with medications for the rest of your life? In order to uncover these truths, it is important to see beyond what we can observe with our five physical senses. The

Bible gives us much greater insights into *why* we struggle with spiritual problems and their resulting diseases, enabling us to perceive beyond what we can see, and to find true healing from disease.

BE IN HEALTH AND FOR MY LIFE

As God opened my eyes to the spiritual roots of disease over thirty years ago, the Be in Health ministry was born. In the beginning, we ministered to people with various diseases on an individual basis and saw them recover. As our journey grew, we began to hold conferences around the world and also created For My Life, inviting people to stay at our Thomaston, Georgia, campus for a one-week, 40-hour retreat. Through these retreats, we have opened our doors to thousands of people, teaching them insights from the Bible and from science to explain why they were sick and God's pathway to healing.[1]

In many ways, our ability to expose the spiritual roots of disease is a direct result of our experiences helping others through For My Life, where we have witnessed countless healings. From conditions as serious as diabetes and cancer to ongoing conditions such as allergies of all kinds, we have seen Father God meet people with healing time and time again. We are grateful to Him for the numerous testimonies we have collected over the years because it is a wonderful reminder that God still honors His Word. However, what is most important are not the physical transformations but the faith and hope that has returned to the hearts of those who have allowed the Holy Spirit to work within them during their time with us.

Because of Father God's love for His creation, He wants to reconnect with His children first, and then heal our bodies as a result. It is God who has inspired our journey and who has worked through me and my team to develop a life-changing ministry to meet anyone seeking healing from disease.

In *Exposing the Spiritual Roots of Disease*, I will describe certain biblical principles through the lens of For My Life so that you may understand how we help people to receive healing and to remain in health. We will uncover

---

1. More recently, we developed For My Life online for those who cannot travel to Georgia because we are determined to help everyone. It is found online through our website, www. BeinHealth.com.

how disease began: what the spiritual roots of disease have been from the beginning, and how they affect us today—in our spirits, our souls, and our bodies. We will expose the unseen forces that trigger disease from within and how we may overcome them.

May I tell you a secret? This book isn't just about exposing the spiritual roots of disease. When people come to us seeking answers, many look disheartened and hopeless, but when they leave, they have a bounce in their step, faith in their hearts, and a renewed excitement to live life again. It isn't just solid Bible teaching that left them with this impression. It is because my team and I care for them—and we care for you, too. I have not dedicated my life to caring for people dying from disease to make a name for myself. It is because Father God loves me, and He loves you. If we are to be healed and made whole, we need to confront the true roots of disease and trust Father God to restore our hearts, our bodies, and our lives.

ONE

DISEASE:
HAPPENSTANCE OR PLANNED EVENT?

Some people think that getting a disease is like standing under the wrong tree at the wrong time and getting hit by random, falling fruit. "Why did this happen to me?" people ask. However, the reason for sickness and disease may not be just a random occurrence.

Why did it happen to you? Why did you get sick? The Christian church and the world look to science and medicine to give them the answers. The truth is that, for many diseases, medicine doesn't have the foggiest idea why they happen. Just like the church, the medical community is at a loss as to how and why many diseases begin. That is why medical books list some diseases with "unknown etiology." As I mentioned earlier, the word etiology refers to origin. It comes from the Greek and means "root cause" or "giving a reason for." "Unknown etiology" simply means, "We don't know the root cause of this disease."

A few of the diseases or syndromes with an unknown etiology include Alzheimer's disease, chronic fatigue syndrome, fibromyalgia, irritable bowel syndrome, and Parkinson's disease. With these illnesses, and others that are considered incurable, the best the medical community can do is to offer "disease management," with a combination of pills, therapies, or surgeries to keep the disease "under control."

Now, you need to know that I am not against doctors; I have been to doctors when necessary. I have spent decades studying what medical science knows about the intricate human body that God has created. But I want to assure you that I do not want to just manage your diseases—I want you to be healed! I stand for disease prevention and eradication, by God's help! I don't want partial relief for you called management. I want to represent your freedom! Why? Because the God I serve—He represents your freedom!

Instead of focusing on medicine and science for why we are sick, I would like to address this question by looking to the wisdom of an ancient text—the Bible. The Bible promises us that Father God will forgive all our iniquities and heal *all* of our diseases. He is the God *"who forgiveth all thine iniquities; who healeth all thy diseases"* (Psalm 103:3).

However, if the Bible gives us the promises of health and healing, why are Christians suffering from diseases like cancer, diabetes, hypertension, Crohn's disease, lupus, depression, and so many more? To find the answer, we are going to take a journey throughout this book. We're going to expose the spiritual roots of disease and discover the way to live in *wholeness*—spirit, soul, and body.

LIVING IN WHOLENESS

What does *wholeness* mean? It is not a "New Age" term. It is our way of describing how God wants us sanctified—wholly, completely. Christians need to understand that we are triune beings. Our foundation comes out of 1 Thessalonians chapter 5, verse 23:

And the very God of peace sanctify you wholly; and I pray God your whole spirit and soul and body be preserved blameless unto the coming of our Lord Jesus Christ. (1 Thessalonians 5:23)

This Scripture does not say we will be sanctified "h-o-l-y," but "w-h-o-l-l-y," or fully, in spirit, soul, and body. In this journey, we will draw the healing of your body together with the health of your soul and spirit.

Why is this important? As a human, you are a spirit, you have a soul, and you live in a body; you are a triune being. Your physical body is like a mobile home. You travel around in it, but often you focus entirely too much energy on it. There's nothing wrong with managing your external house. After all, we paint our homes, put shutters on them, plant flowers around them, and enjoy their beauty. But the truth is, the real you is not your physical body, no matter how much "poly-plastic" or Mary Kay makeup you may use! We have become the product of our five physical senses!

Through Be in Health, we have ministered to people from around the world who have some understanding of their *spirit* (the part if us that is eternal) from their churches and the Bible, some understanding about their *soul* (our mind, will, and emotions) from psychologists, and some understanding about their *body* from medical doctors. What they don't understand is that we are impacted by more than what we perceive externally. We are also impacted from within, at the spirit level. The pivotal role that Be in Health and the For My Life retreats play is to draw all three—spirit, soul, and body—together. We must learn the truth of how the enemy attacks the whole man—spirit, soul, and body.

WHAT IS THE ROOT OF DISEASE?

So, what is the root cause of disease? I want to make it clear from the very beginning that I believe the root cause of 80 percent of disease is spiritual and is the result of separation on three levels:

1. Separation from Father God—from His person, His love, and His Word.

2. Separation from yourself.

3. Separation from others.

You need to follow this closely because these separations are the spiritual root of so many diseases that plague us. If 80 percent of all disease involves these separations, then 80 percent of all healing begins with reconciliation to God, reconciliation to yourself, and reconciliation to others. Let me repeat: *the beginning of healing starts with the restoration of your relationship with God, yourself, and others.*

SEPARATION FROM FATHER GOD

Mankind is diseased first of all because we are separated from Father God, His Word, and His love. This is the most troubling area of separation. At Be in Health, we have discovered that in the healing and prevention of disease, it is important that we resolve our issues with our heavenly Father.

Over the years, speaking to Christians from all walks of life, we have found that many people feel much closer to Jesus than they do to the Father. Jesus is their Savior, who took all their sins upon Himself, so they are confident of His love. But they don't feel the same connection with Father God, who may seem so much farther away in heavenly places or who may seem like a "taskmaster" waiting for them to make a mistake. However, that is not what the truth of God's Word tells us. The Bible tells us that God is love: *"And we have known and believed the love that God hath to us. God is love; and he that dwelleth in love dwelleth in God, and God in him"* (1 John 4:16).

Do you believe the Father would have sent His Son to die for us if He didn't love us? If He was an angry God who was looking to punish us? The reason Jesus came to earth was to reconcile us to the Father. He came to show us the Father and His love for us. Jesus showed us the deep love of the Father by dying on the cross for our eternal redemption.

Philip saith unto him, Lord, show us the Father, and it sufficeth us. Jesus saith unto him, Have I been so long time with you, and yet hast thou not known me, Philip? he that hath seen me hath seen the Father; and how sayest thou then, Show us the Father? (John 14:8–9)

Perhaps, as Christians, we do not always feel safe with God as our Father because of the many issues we have with our earthly fathers. Many people associate God the Father with the failure of an earthly father, and then our heavenly Father is guilty by association. (It is important that you also resolve any issues with your earthly father, because some of you weren't properly cared for by your earthly father. That will be addressed in a later chapter.)

If Jesus came to show us the Father, and your earthly father didn't represent Him, may I introduce you to your true Father?

+ Because of His love for you, God chose to make you His son or daughter. You didn't go looking for Him; He came looking for you, and you responded. As it says in John 1:12, *"But as many as received him, to them gave he power to become the sons of God, even to them that believe on his name."* In 2 Corinthians 6:18, we read, *"And [I] will be a Father unto you, and ye shall be my sons and daughters, saith the Lord Almighty.*

+ Every good thing that you can think of in your life came to you from your heavenly Father. *"Every good gift and every perfect gift is from above, and cometh down from the Father of lights, with whom is no variableness, neither shadow of turning"* (James 1:17).

+ Because of Jesus's sacrifice on the cross, you have been adopted into God's family. He has given you the privilege to cry out to Him, "Abba Father," which means "Daddy"! *"For ye have not received the spirit of bondage again to fear; but ye have received the Spirit of adoption, whereby we cry, Abba, Father"* (Romans 8:15).

When we look at ourselves, do we truly believe that we were created to be a reflection of Father God on earth, or do we view ourselves through the lens of past failure and years of shame and guilt? To be reconciled to God, we need to repent of having believed Satan's lies against us and embrace the truth of the Father's love for us according to the Bible.

To be free and healed, you must believe God's Word that He truly loves you in spite of a lifetime of failures that may suggest otherwise. After all, you were not saved because of your own righteousness but because of the gift of eternal life paid for by Jesus Christ at the cross.

As we continue our study of the root causes of disease, believe that the Father desires health and wholeness for you. Accept Father God's great love for you; He has called you to be His own! As He says in Jeremiah 31:3, *"Yea, I have loved thee with an everlasting love: therefore with lovingkindness have I drawn thee."*

SEPARATION FROM OURSELVES

In addition to the disease caused by separation from the Father, *separation from ourselves* is also a foundational part of our observations. For decades, we have ministered to thousands of people who have battled intensely with self-hatred, self-loathing, self-bitterness, and guilt. They have been told by loved ones, or by thoughts in their heads planted by Satan, that they have no value. Every failure and mistake proves to them that they are unlovable. These are deep-rooted lies from the enemy that carry with them many disorders, especially autoimmune diseases. Additionally, if we believe we are junk, it is a sure sign that we do not understand the love Father God has for us.

If this is your struggle, you must learn to set down those lies and repent to Father God of having believed them. If He doesn't view you through the lens of your past failures, you must learn to repent for judging yourself by them in defiance of His love toward you. You are being called to resist the deception of self-hatred and guilt. Do not forget, God loves you! He declares it in His Word. Do not deny the truth of His love for you by believing the lies of the enemy. At For My Life, we dedicate many hours to comparing Scriptures to the lies of Satan's kingdom. When retreat attendees recognize the lies and repent to Father God, many of them are healed.

SEPARATION FROM OTHERS

Finally, *separation from others* opens the door to many spiritually rooted diseases. The Word cautions us: *"Looking diligently lest any man fail of the grace of God; lest any root of bitterness springing up trouble you, and thereby many be defiled"* (Hebrews 12:15).

Unforgiveness and bitterness can become a root deep inside of you that defiles those around you and makes your body very susceptible to disease. It is your choice alone to make peace with your father, your mother, your sibling, the church, and anyone else who has injured you. You are not responsible for what other people think about you, but you are responsible to forgive them for any injury done to you. Perhaps someone is unwilling to talk to you, or they have passed away. If you cannot repent to them, you can still be free of sin. However, you are responsible for forgiving them from your heart and repenting to Father God for bitterness despite what they have done to you even if you cannot have face-to-face closure with them. If you repent to Father God for bitterness, He will forgive you, and that is what counts. *"If we confess our sins, he is faithful and just to forgive us our sins, and to cleanse us from all unrighteousness"* (1 John 1:9).

When we are separated from God, ourselves, and others, we are following the enemy's plan for humankind. His goal is to cause our destruction. As Jesus explained it, *"The thief cometh not, but for to steal, and to kill, and to destroy: I am come that they might have life, and that they might have it more abundantly"* (John 10:10).

When we embrace the enemy's lies, we end up suffering at his hands. The Bible warns us not to be *"ignorant of* [Satan's] *devices"*: *"Lest Satan should get an advantage of us: for we are not ignorant of his devices"* (2 Corinthians 2:11).

That word *"devices"* means methods or practices—the ways he tries to destroy. You need to know how the enemy causes separation and sin. You need to understand his devices so that you can cut him off at the pass in your life! Let's consider where Satan's devices against humankind began.

WHERE DID SEPARATION AND DISEASE BEGIN?

Do you know how many diseases there are? Over three thousand disorders and diseases have been identified! Where did they all come from? They didn't come from God. When He created man, Father God created something that was very good, but then something came along to interfere, something that wasn't good at all. In order to understand the spiritual roots of disease, we need to lay some groundwork for how sin and disease entered our world.

In the book of Luke, Jesus said He saw Satan fall from heaven. *"And he said unto them, I beheld Satan as lightning fall from heaven"* (Luke 10:18).

I have done extensive teachings about the fall of Lucifer, or Heylel (phonetic translation of the Hebrew), but this is not my main topic. My point is that he was a covering cherub before he fell and rebelled against God. He also took a third of the angels with him. After he "fell from heaven," he was known as Satan, translated from the Greek as "the Accuser." That is a fitting title for him because he has impugned the character of God to humans and led us to act against our Creator. I believe these events took place before the events of the garden of Eden and that is how he took the form of a serpent to speak to Adam and Eve.

Let's take a look at Genesis, chapters 2 and 3—the creation of Adam and Eve, their relationship with Father God, and their fall. How long were Adam and Eve in the garden of Eden before they fell? We don't know for certain. Some people think it all happened in just one day: Adam was created in the morning, Eve was brought alongside at noon, they were tempted by afternoon, and they fell in the evening. However, the Bible never tells us how long Adam and Eve walked with God. They could have been in the garden for as long as a thousand years.

Why am I pointing this out? The account of Genesis is not just about the mechanical order of creation. Instead, it is the account of the Godhead—Father, Son, and Holy Spirit—and their love for us—their creation. The Lord spent time with Adam and cared for him. He did not just care about Adam's physical needs. He cared about his relational needs, as well. It was the Lord who recognized Adam needed a partner. God created Eve for Adam so he would not be alone. The Lord was not withdrawn from His creation but wished to fellowship with them. In fact, even after Adam and Eve fell into sin, the Lord came into the garden to talk with them.

And they heard the voice of the Lord *God walking in the garden in the cool of the day: and Adam and his wife hid themselves from the presence of the* Lord *God amongst the trees of the garden.*

(Genesis 3:8)

In order to understand exactly why Adam and Eve fell, we need to understand that instructions were given to Adam, but he disobeyed God's commandment. According to the second chapter of Genesis, just before Eve was created, Adam was given the first commandment from God.

And the Lord *God commanded the man, saying, Of every tree of the garden thou mayest freely eat: but of the tree of the knowledge of good*

and evil, thou shalt not eat of it: for in the day that thou eatest thereof
thou shalt surely die.   (Genesis 2:16–17)

Was that rule so difficult to memorize? It was a mere two verses long! "That tree over there—that fruit? Don't eat the fruit. Because the day that you eat the fruit, you will surely die." Maybe Adam didn't communicate those lines very well to Eve. We know that Adam and Eve disobeyed that first commandment of God. Then came spiritual death, or separation from God because of sin.

SATAN, THE GREAT DECEIVER

When Satan tempted Eve in the garden of Eden, he revealed one of his strongest devices—Satan changed the Word of God: *"Now the serpent was more subtil than any beast of the field which the* LORD *God had made. And he said unto the woman, Yea, hath God said, Ye shall not eat of every tree of the garden?"* (Genesis 3:1).

After Eve responded that there was only one tree that they couldn't eat from, Satan challenged God's Word again. *"And the serpent said unto the woman, Ye shall not surely die: for God doth know that in the day ye eat thereof, then your eyes shall be opened, and ye shall be as gods, knowing good and evil"* (Genesis 3:4–5).

Satan willfully added *to* and subtracted *from* God's words. He said that God didn't really say they would die, but they would become as "gods." The King James Version translators did an excellent job translating the term "gods." Contrary to what some may believe, it is not capital "G," God, but lowercase "g," gods. If they ate of the fruit in disobedience to God's commandment, they would not replace God but operate as "gods." What does that mean? It actually means they would become as "devils." Satan's kingdom is purposely set against the knowledge of God to bring us into captivity to its ways by deception. Adam and Eve were deceived into believing they would be their own gods. They were brought under the bondage of Satan and his kingdom instead.

As soon as Adam partook of the fruit, their spiritual eyes were opened, and at that moment, evil flooded in. When their eyes were opened, they saw their nakedness, perceived it as unclean, and were ashamed. Adam and Eve had enjoyed close fellowship with God, but now they were afraid of Him. Adam, a son of God, was suddenly afraid of the One whom he had always walked with in the cool of the evening.

As evening approached, it was time for the Lord to meet with them. Adam turned to his wife and said, "It's time for the Lord. Look at us. We are so evil. Let's go hide." So, they ran and hid in the bushes. The Lord came looking for them, and they weren't there. He called out, "Where are you, Adam?" Finally, Adam had enough nerve to answer, "Here we are, Lord!" "Where, Adam?" "Out here in the bushes." "Why are you out there in the bushes, Adam?" "Hiding from You, Lord." "Why are you hiding from Me, Adam?" "Because, Lord, we are naked."

Now, consider the words of the Lord in Genesis 3:11: *"And he said, Who told thee that thou wast naked? Hast thou eaten of the tree, whereof I commanded thee that thou shouldest not eat?"*

Why did God ask Adam, "Who told you?" Because God knew why Adam and Eve were hiding, and He also knew the answer to His question. He knew it was Satan who had interfered with His perfect creation with the sole aim of bringing destruction—sin, separation from God, and death. He knew who was giving Adam and Eve thoughts of fear, guilt, and shame. God identified Adam's thoughts and feelings as coming from Satan's deceptive kingdom. But God wanted Adam to recognize, as well, that the thoughts he had were not his own; they came from a separate being.

We should note here that the Lord did not ask Adam what he felt or what he was thinking about during the temptation. God did not ask Adam about his feelings. When Jesus was tempted in the wilderness, did He check with His feelings or rationalize with Satan about the validity of Satan's temptations? No! The way Jesus defeated Satan's lies was by quoting the Word of God back to him. Perhaps, instead of trying to discern good and evil for ourselves, we need to return to what the Bible has said must be our standard.

Then was Jesus led up of the Spirit into the wilderness to be tempted of the devil. And when he had fasted forty days and forty nights, he was afterward an hungred. And when the tempter came to him, he said, If thou be the Son of God, command that these stones be made bread. But he answered and said, It is written, Man shall not live by bread alone, but by every word that proceedeth out of the mouth of God.

(Matthew 4:1–4)

Jesus overcame two more temptations in the wilderness with God's Word. We need to learn to defeat Satan's lies in the same way.

IT IS A PLANNED EVENT

None of the separation, sin, and disease that mankind has experienced since the garden of Eden is a happenstance or accident. It is all a planned event against us by the villain, Satan, and his kingdom. By failing to address Satan's kingdom and its influence over our life, thoughts, and behavior, we fail to address a major reason why we are diseased and tormented. Much of the Christian church has somehow forgotten the enemy who is after our destruction—spirit, soul, and body. The church has forgotten that we need discernment from God to wage a spiritual war against that enemy and to expose him for who he is—the destroyer.

The good news is that you and I have the ability to discern good from evil. Discernment does not come by instinct; it is a gift of the Holy Spirit. Discerning the true reason behind disease is available to us through God's Word. With the truth of the Word, we will overcome this planned event called *disease* and live the healthy and long lives God has promised us. *Freedom from disease can be ours.*

The Godhead has brought us the truth found in the Bible. It brings freedom by sanctifying our spirit, our soul, and our body. It is my desire that this journey of knowledge we are taking will fill you with God's truth and peace and produce the understanding and wisdom that will set you free from all manner of disease.

SPIRITUAL WARFARE AND THE CHURCH

The result of Adam and Eve's fall was that sin, death, and disease entered the world. And a spiritual battle between the kingdom of God and the kingdom of Satan began for the hearts and minds of mankind. The Bible is clear that our battle is not against flesh and blood:

> For we wrestle not against flesh and blood, but against principalities, against powers, against the rulers of the darkness of this world, against spiritual wickedness in high places.   (Ephesians 6:12)

Please understand, your war is not with other humans. Your war is not even with yourselves. Your war is with an invisible, evil kingdom ruled by principalities, powers, the rulers of the darkness of this world, and spiritual wickedness in high places. Because that kingdom is invisible, our war is primarily with thoughts and feelings we act upon that contradict the Word of God.

The spirit world is a place where intelligent beings exist that do not have bodies in the physical sense. There are two parts of this invisible world, two kingdoms. There's the part that the Father rules, which is the kingdom of God, or heaven. Heaven is not far away; it's in a different dimension, just on the other side of what we can see. There is another kingdom in the spirit world that is inhabited by fallen beings that are ruled by Satan. That kingdom is clearly identified in the Bible as well. Jesus spoke of it on more than one occasion. In Matthew 12:26, He said, *"And if Satan cast out Satan, he is divided against himself; how shall then his kingdom stand?"*

We need to understand the warfare between these two kingdoms. In the military, soldiers are trained for combat; they are trained to *know* their enemy and to utilize the weapons and tactics needed to defeat him. Our challenge is that the weapons of our warfare against our enemy are not carnal; they are spiritual. What is carnal? The physical world and all physical weapons are carnal; they are things we can see and touch. But *"the weapons of our warfare are not carnal, but mighty through God to the pulling down of strong holds"* (2 Corinthians 10:4).

Just as it was for Adam, our war is with an enemy who wants to form us into his image. By becoming bitter, fearful, or disheartened, we will think, speak, and act like Satan and his kingdom—this is the image of death. When we choose to love, forgive, and operate according to the instructions of the Bible, we are following after Christ. The image of death is what Adam and Eve embraced. We must learn to embrace life.

So, what are we to do? We need to receive spiritual training. We need to develop discernment according to Scripture. Without this knowledge, the Christian church will remain in the dark ages when it comes to understanding the spiritual roots of disease. Hosea 4:6 warns us: *"My people are destroyed for lack of knowledge."*

God's people are suffering because they don't have the knowledge that they need to be in health. I did a brief language study of these words in Hosea. When God says, *"My people are destroyed,"* it's actually in the progressive present tense: "my people *are being* destroyed for lack of knowledge." If the people of God are being destroyed, in the present, then this warning is not just for the Old Testament believers. The New Testament church is also currently being destroyed. I see this same lack of knowledge in the modern church. However, I am not your accuser.

I deal with New Testament saints who have diseases. I deal with New Testament saints who have issues of the soul. I deal with New Testament saints who have serious problems. And, for many of them, I know why. You need to know why, as well. That's what this book is all about.

So, how do we return to correct knowledge and understanding? We turn to the Bible for God's truth.

WHAT IS TRUTH?

In today's world, even in some parts of the Christian church, there is the perception that truth is "relative." Opinions in the church and the world constitute a sort of framework of belief based upon personal observations and "feelings." The Bible clearly tells us that truth is in the Scriptures, it is God-inspired, and it is not open to personal interpretation. Second Timothy 3:16 explains, *"All scripture is given by inspiration of God, and is profitable for doctrine, for reproof, for correction, for instruction in righteousness."* And we read in 2 Peter 1:20, *"Knowing this first, that no prophecy of the scripture is of any private interpretation."*

So, why does much of the church and world doubt the truth of the Word of God? If the truth of Scripture is incontrovertible, where is the proof of changed lives and the miraculous in the world today? Why are so many sons and daughters of Father God suffering from as much disease as the world? Why do we have the same biological diseases, the same psychiatric problems? Could it be that many supposed teachings suggesting the end of miracles and healing are the result of incorrect doctrine and not a failure of Scripture to fulfill the promises of God?

It is time to reinvestigate the Scriptures. It is time to take a closer look at the truth of God's Word. We often tell our attendees at For My Life that we may touch your "sacred cows" of belief, but if we only regurgitate conventional Christian beliefs without conclusive proof from the Bible, we will be left with the same mess we see in the church and the world today.

THE FULLNESS OF GOD'S WORD

The Bible is the Word of God. The Scriptures promising wholeness and healing are key examples of the love of the Father and His desire to see us whole. For example, Psalm 103:2–3 says, *"Bless the LORD, O my soul, and forget not all his benefits: who forgiveth all thine iniquities; who healeth all thy diseases."*

Faith in God and in His Word is vital to your journey of health and healing. But let me ask you a question: Are you willing to accept the *fullness* of God's Word? Perhaps we have been striving with an increased emphasis on faith without balancing it against repentance from sin in our lives. The same Bible full of God's promises also contains warnings about following after sin and Satan's kingdom. If we believe the promises of God are incontrovertible, should we not also fully accept that the consequences of sin also carry a price? *"Know ye not, that to whom ye yield yourselves servants to obey, his servants ye are to whom ye obey; whether of sin unto death, or of obedience unto righteousness?"* (Romans 6:16).

What we have found over years of ministering the Word of God is the importance of preaching *repentance from dead works* along with faith toward God. Do you realize that faith toward God is the second doctrine of Christ? Many in the church teach it as the first and only doctrine of Christ, but according to the Scriptures, the first doctrine is repentance from dead works. Perhaps what hinders our faith and our healing from disease is *not* addressing the stumbling block of sin in our lives before assessing faith in our lives.

> *Therefore leaving the principles of the doctrine of Christ, let us go on unto perfection; not laying again the foundation of repentance from dead works, and of faith toward God, of the doctrine of baptisms, and of laying on of hands, and of resurrection of the dead, and of eternal judgment.* (Hebrews 6:1–2)

THE IMPACT OF OUR SPIRITUALITY

Have you ever considered that living a life perpetually offended and bitter or stressed out can be bad for your body? How about the fact that the Bible specifically instructs you against such lifestyles? Have you ever considered that your spirituality (spirit) impacts the way you think (soul) and, in turn, impacts the way your body functions? By looking at our spirituality, we have found that recognizing and repenting of sin will produce peaceable thoughts and healing for our bodies. *"Looking diligently lest any man fail of the grace of God; lest any root of bitterness springing up trouble you, and thereby many be defiled"* (Hebrews 12:15).

Why does the church struggle with the connection of sin and disease? Did Jesus fail to show us the Father correctly? Of course not. Then where is the disconnect?

A major reason why we struggle with disease is this idea of addressing sin in our lives. Many Christians avoid reading their Bible because they feel as if God is condemning them for sinning. They do not feel like they can measure up to the Scriptures. In some segments of Christianity, they believe grace is a cover for sin. As correctly defined by *Strong's Exhaustive Concordance*, the Greek definition of grace is "divine influence upon the heart, and its reflection in the life."[2] It is not a license to sin without

---

2. *Charis*, Greek #4385 in Strong's *Exhaustive Concordance*, Bible Hub, https://biblehub.com/greek/5485.htm.

consequences. If you drive on the wrong side of the road, do you really expect not to get in a car crash?

Sin is much the same way. If we follow after Satan's kingdom of lies, if we follow after unrighteousness, shouldn't we expect consequences? In other words, should we sin more that grace might more abound? God forbid. *"What shall we say then? Shall we continue in sin, that grace may abound? God forbid. How shall we, that are dead to sin, live any longer therein?"* (Romans 6:1–2).

Unfortunately, too many in the church wrongly conclude that repentance is only for unbelievers and *not* for Christians. They want to be blessed and healthy and yet live in sin. The problem is that sin is making them unhealthy. You can scour the internet to find ample evidence from medical science that living a bitter or stressed-out/fearful lifestyle has been linked to many physical and psychological conditions. If you wish to remain bitter and angry, but expect to have a healthy mind and body, even medical science cannot guarantee you a positive result. The reason, as we will continue to explore, is because anger and bitterness may in fact be the root issue making your body diseased.

RESTORING YOU BACK TO HEALTH

As you'll learn throughout *Exposing the Spiritual Roots of Disease*, the key roots of many diseases are elements of Satan's kingdom: bitterness, accusation, envy and jealousy, fear, anxiety and stress, anger and hostility, rejection, shame, unloving spirits, self-hate, occultism, and addictions. The purpose of sin is not just to make you feel bad. These sin issues are planned events by the enemy. They are destructive to you, your relationships, and Father God's plan for your life.

My little children, these things write I unto you, that ye sin not. And if any man sin, we have an advocate with the Father, Jesus Christ the righteous: and he is the propitiation for our sins: and not for ours only, but also for the sins of the whole world. (1 John 2:1–2)

At For My Life, we routinely see people healed of various physical and psychological diseases once they recognize areas of their life where they have served Satan's kingdom and sin, and repent to God without anyone praying over them. The work of my lifetime is to pass on the truth about these spiritual roots of disease to as many people as I can—to share the logic and heart behind the formation of For My Life, and our mission to work with Father God to restore humanity back to health and, as a result, back to His heart.

My desire is to open your eyes to God's truth concerning freedom from disease. I want you to walk in freedom. I want you to defeat everything that God hates. Satan may have his devices or tactics, but God will show you how you can defeat him and be in health. You should be a thriver! While the world might be struggling in disease and hopelessness, you should be a happy, well-balanced, and enthusiastic son or daughter of God.

TWO

IS DISEASE A BLESSING OR A CURSE?

One of the saddest moments in my ministry was when I came upon a man struggling with a disease. He was a believer, and I asked him if he would like prayer to be healed. He turned me down by remarking that God had given him his disease. His erroneous belief led him to reject the potential of healing.

Over the years, we have found many people who believe Satan's lie that God has given them their diseases. It has led them to a place of torment because they are confused as to whether God wants them to live or die. At our For My Life retreats, it is important that we define blessings and curses to help the attendees reevaluate what they have come to believe. It may very well be the difference between life and death for many of them! Many are healed during the week when they understand that God did not give them disease; His desire is for them to be healed and whole instead!

If some Christians truly believe disease is from God, then why do they seek medical treatment for their conditions? If disease is a blessing from God, why would you interfere with His will for your life? Because of how much damage this erroneous position has caused, it is essential we disprove it. If the Bible reveals disease is evil and a curse, then it is impossible that God would give us diseases. This verse in the book of James clearly states God does not tempt us with evil, nor can He be tempted with it: *"Let no man say when he is tempted, I am tempted of God: for God cannot be tempted with evil, neither tempteth he any man"* (James 1:13).

In order to establish biblical truth on blessings and curses, it is important to begin in the Old Testament. Nearing the end of his long life, Moses stood before an audience of hundreds of thousands of Israelites, just as he had done countless times before. God had given him some critical things to say to His people on how they should live once they entered the promised land without Moses as their guide. They had better listen carefully! The message was also a warning. God was offering them a clear choice between blessings and curses, between health and disease. *"I call heaven and earth to record this day against you, that I have set before you life and death, blessing and cursing: therefore choose life, that both thou and thy seed may live"* (Deuteronomy 30:19).

Moses gives us the details of these blessings and curses in Deuteronomy 28. He reveals God's truth that we all need to know concerning the spiritual roots of disease.

And it shall come to pass, if thou shalt hearken diligently unto the voice of the LORD *thy God, to observe and to do all his commandments which I command thee this day, that the* LORD *thy God will set thee on high above all nations of the earth: and all these blessings shall come on thee, and overtake thee, if thou shalt hearken unto the voice of the* LORD *thy God.* (Deuteronomy 28:1–2)

Look what God is promising! His people will be *"high above all nations of the earth,"* and they will receive more blessings than they can count! In the next twelve verses, Moses delivers a list of blessings that will *"overtake"* them: blessings in their cities and in their countryside, blessings in their families and in their fields, blessings in their battles and in their health. Moses says the blessings will not only follow them but will also overtake them, if they will only listen and obey the Lord. What a promise! If they will only listen and obey. But Moses's message doesn't end there. He follows with a warning that he never wants them to forget. Here is God's Word from the opposite side of the coin:

> *But it shall come to pass, if thou wilt not hearken unto the voice of the*
> *Lord thy God, to observe to do all his commandments and his statutes*
> *which I command thee this day; that all these curses shall come upon*
> *thee, and overtake thee.*   (Deuteronomy 28:15)

For the next forty-three verses, Moses describes the curses—the disastrous events and the diseases—that will overtake God's chosen people if they choose not to listen to Him and refuse to follow His commandments. By their disobedience, they will open themselves up to curses...and many of those curses are diseases.

Be assured, God is not behind the consequences of disobedience to His Word. Instead, He wants you to make the right choices. Later in Deuteronomy, chapter 30, Moses, as God's representative, clearly implores the Israelites to choose life. Father God wants you to choose life too. *"I call heaven and earth to record this day against you, that I have set before you life and death, blessing and cursing: therefore choose life, that both thou and thy seed may live"* (Deuteronomy 30:19–20).

IS MOSES'S MESSAGE PROPHETIC?

In Deuteronomy 28:1, Moses declares, *"And it shall come to pass...."*

> *And it shall come to pass, if thou shalt hearken diligently unto the voice*
> *of the Lord thy God, to observe and to do all his commandments*
> *which I command thee this day, that the Lord thy God will set thee on*
> *high above all nations of the earth.*   (Deuteronomy 28:1)

Is that prophetic? It sure is! There is no statement in the Bible any more prophetic than *"It shall come to pass."* Now, is this prophetic promise also conditional? Yes, it is. Nobody wants to make anything conditional these days, but God has conditions. He sets the standard, and it is our responsibility to respond to the standard. *"These blessings shall come on thee, and overtake thee, if thou shalt hearken unto the voice of the Lord thy God"* (Deuteronomy 28:2).

Let's look at the word "*if*" used in these Bible passages. Deuteronomy 28:2 begins to describe the blessings that will result from obedience to God's Word: "*And all these blessings shall come on thee, and overtake thee, if thou shalt hearken unto the voice of the LORD thy God.*"

The key to this verse is the Hebrew word for "*if*" used here. It is roughly translated phonetically as "kiy" or" "kee." The implication of this word from *Strong's Concordance* is a "causal connection."[3] It is cause and effect. *If* you follow the Word of God, you will surely be blessed by God. There is a surety of conclusion because the promises of God are definite.

However, in verse 15, when Moses repeats the words "*it shall come to pass,*" he uses a different Hebrew word for "*if*": "*But it shall come to pass, if thou wilt not hearken unto the voice of the LORD thy God, to observe to do all his commandments and his statutes which I command thee this day; that all these curses shall come upon thee, and overtake thee*" (Deuteronomy 28:15).

This time, the word "*if*" is translated from the Hebrew phonetically as "im" or "eem." It is conditional in the definition provided by *Strong's*.[4] This "*if*" serves as a warning for believers. *If* you do not listen to the Lord and you go another way, curses will come upon you and overtake you. This form of the word "*if*" indicates it moves slower because of the mercy of God. It offers a place to change course so that curses do not come upon you.

God is full of mercy. Don't feel condemned by sin. Repent to Him and receive blessings instead! One thing I want you to understand: I am not advocating a return to the law of Moses. I am not into legalism. I am into something called heart change! I am into understanding the fullness of God's Word because it is truth, and that truth brings us freedom from disease.

WHAT EXACTLY IS A CURSE?

God said that if His people disobeyed His commandments, curses would overtake them. But what, exactly, is a curse?

---

3. *Strong's* Hebrew #3588, Bible Hub, https://biblehub.com/strongs/deuteronomy/28-2.htm.
4. *Strong's* Hebrew #518, Bible Hub, https://biblehub.com/strongs/deuteronomy/28-15.htm.

In the church I grew up in, people believed that the word *curse* existed in the Old Testament but not in the New Testament. Maybe you have had the same experience. Yet, when I looked at all the things that were called "curses" in the Old Testament and realized that many New Testament saints had the same problems in their lives, I began to reexamine the meaning of a curse.

Every class of disease known to man is found in those verses of Deuteronomy 28, and God called them the result of a curse. That includes everything right down to hemorrhoids, insanity, anxiety disorders, and torment. I saw that these same diseases were plaguing far too many believers today. Believers had autoimmune disorders; they had depression; they had incurable diseases. In the morning, they wished to God it were night, and at nighttime, they wished to God it were morning.

In the morning thou shalt say, Would God it were even! and at even thou shalt say, Would God it were morning! for the fear of thine heart wherewith thou shalt fear, and for the sight of thine eyes which thou shalt see. (Deuteronomy 28:67)

These believers were filled with fear and torment, and they had all kinds of disorders. I thought to myself, "Why have these psychological and biological disorders—called curses in the Old Testament, also found in New Testament believers— cease to be called curses any longer?"

During our Be in Health conferences, I asked other Christians, "Why aren't diseases considered a curse today?" Their answer was often, "They're just a disease." Some churches were more adamant, stating that curses no longer exist. In these audiences, I had to phrase it differently: "Are diseases a blessing or a 'blank'?" I couldn't use the word "curse," so I used the word "blank"!

DOES GOD SEND CURSES?

Does God send curses to us? Some people point to Paul's "thorn in the flesh" as coming from God, but there is a problem with presuming this position. Why? This thorn is known as a "messenger of Satan." *"And lest I should be exalted above measure through the abundance of the revelations, there was given to me a thorn in the flesh, the messenger of Satan to buffet me, lest I should be exalted above measure"* (2 Corinthians 12:7).

I have a very serious concern about anyone insisting that God purposely and actively sent this messenger to Paul. Why? Because of James, chapter 1. God doesn't tempt man with any kind of evil, including "messengers of Satan." The messenger was not from God but from Satan. *"Let no man say when he is tempted, I am tempted of God: for God cannot be tempted with evil, neither tempteth he any man"* (James 1:13).

If Father God gave Paul this "thorn," then why would He also strengthen him in the midst of it? The answer is God did not give it to him; instead, Father God was making a provision for Paul to overcome it. *"And he said unto me, My grace is sufficient for thee: for my strength is made perfect in weakness. Most gladly therefore will I rather glory in my infirmities, that the power of Christ may rest upon me"* (2 Corinthians 12:9).

Paul had a problem, and God wanted him to overcome it. Father God did not give him a "messenger from Satan," but, as we will see later, Paul tells us that he has some sin in his life that made him susceptible to Satan's kingdom. As the book of James puts it, we are tempted when we are "drawn away of our own lust": *"But every man is tempted, when he is drawn away of his own lust, and enticed"* (James 1:14).

Have you ever wondered why different people have different addictions or other weaknesses of character? Some people are fearful. Some people are angry. Some people are bitter. It is because each person, their family, and their generations have a different weakness that can lead to sin. As a result, we teach on a diversity of topics, from fear to bitterness to accusation and others, because we recognize we all struggle in different ways.

I realize many in Christianity have a philosophy of why disease isn't a curse, and they are the first ones to argue about this. However, as we minister to hurting people, our team is faced with difficult situations all the time. Should we tell people tormented with sin that God wants them to die of cancer or to live with depression forever? No. We help them uncover the roots of why they have these curses in their lives and help them identify where they have a spiritual weakness so they may recover. God is the one who meets them with healing and restoration, often without prayer from us. He is not the one creating the problem, but He is the one providing the solution!

WHAT DOES A CURSE DO?

I decided to do a little study of the Hebrew word curse based on Deuteronomy 28. You can do it, too, with a copy of *Strong's Concordance*. The first word I found for the meaning of curse was *vilification*. What in the world? I went to God and asked, "Sir, *curse* in the Hebrew is defined as 'vilification.' What does that mean?"

God answered, "Henry, you know how to break the word down to its roots." Okay! Vilification starts with the same letters as the word *villain*. The minute I saw the word *villain*, a Scripture from the New Testament sprang into my consciousness. That Scripture was John 10:10: *"The thief cometh not, but for to steal, and to kill, and to destroy: I am come that they might have life, and that they might have it more abundantly."*

That thief, Satan, is the enemy, the villain in our lives. Then I drilled further down in the word study, and I ran across this: a curse is the abatement of the blessing. The word *abatement* means "lessening" or "reduction." So, the villain, who is Satan, comes to abate, reduce, or take away the strength of our blessings from God. The curse is the work of this villain. Vilification is when the villain vilifies or reduces our blessings!

WHEN CAN A CURSE AFFECT A CHRISTIAN?

This brings up a new question: "How do curses affect Christians today?" The Bible tells us that a curse without cause, or without a reason for being there, cannot affect us. We read in Proverbs 26:2, *"As the bird by wandering, as the swallow by flying, so the curse causeless shall not come."* And in Galatians 3:13, it says, *"Christ hath redeemed us from the curse of the law, being made a curse for us: for it is written, Cursed is every one that hangeth on a tree."*

Didn't Christ end the curse brought on mankind by Adam and Eve through His death on the cross? Yes, He did. And by His death and resurrection, He made it possible for us to live in righteousness and wholeness. However, continuing in sin is how Christians, who are covered by the blood of the Lamb, can be under the burden of a curse. The effects of the curse are a result of disobedience to God's Word, and Christians can be just as disobedient to God's Word as Old Testament believers were! Curses can come because we give them permission to do it!

The problem with the word *curse* is that many people base their understanding of it upon movies, television, and superstition. Now, I am not talking about Christians being possessed by an evil spirit like the Gadarene demoniac. I am not talking about losing your salvation. I am talking about servitude to the enemy. I am talking about serving the law of sin rather than the law of God. How do we do that? As one example, when the Bible instructs us to forgive, and we choose to remain bitter over past transgressions done against us, we are choosing to serve sin in that area. The result of choosing Satan's lies over God's Word can be very damaging.

A curse that has no cause cannot affect a Christian. But a curse can affect us if we give the villain who is behind that curse permission to wreak havoc in our lives. Satan doesn't have all power. He can only touch us with our permission. How do we give the devil this permission? *By disobeying God and His Word and obeying the law of sin instead.*

PAUL'S WAR WITH SIN

In Romans, chapter 7, the apostle Paul explains that there is a war raging within each of us between following God's Word and following the law of sin. Even though Paul was a committed follower of Christ, he confessed that there was a war within him, with two laws battling for his soul: the law of God and the law of sin.

> For the good that I would I do not: but the evil which I would not, that I do. Now if I do that I would not, it is no more I that do it, but sin that dwelleth in me. I find then a law, that, when I would do good, evil is present with me. For I delight in the law of God after the inward man: but I see another law in my members, warring against the law of my mind, and bringing me into captivity to the law of sin which is in my

members. O wretched man that I am! who shall deliver me from the body of this death? I thank God through Jesus Christ our Lord. So then with the mind I myself serve the law of God; but with the flesh the law of sin. (Romans 7:19–25)

This battle of the law of sin against the law of God that happened within Paul still happens in us today. Don't tell me that you aren't tempted by the law of sin or that you are stronger than Paul in overcoming temptation! The law of sin comes to each one of us to compete with the law of God.

What is the law of God? "I thought we weren't under the law of Moses," you might question again. When Paul talks about the law of God, he is referring to God's nature. The law is a reflection of God's righteousness. God is good; God is love; God is justice; God is forgiveness; God is faithfulness. These things and more are His nature and His righteousness. His nature is the law that God promises to write on our hearts. As the psalmist put it, *"I delight to do thy will, O my God: yea, thy law is within my heart"* (Psalm 40:8). And in Hebrews 8:10, it says, *"For this is the covenant that I will make with the house of Israel after those days, saith the Lord; I will put my laws into their mind, and write them in their hearts: and I will be to them a God, and they shall be to me a people."*

THE LAW OF SIN

On the other side of the war, the nature of Satan is found under the category of the law of sin: rebellion, lawlessness, falsehoods, hatred, murder, evil. The law of sin will always attempt to fall upon us to compete with the law of God. As Paul said, "The things that I wish I wouldn't do, that's what I do. The things I hate, I do, and the good that I want to do, I don't do." Well, that sounds just like us, doesn't it?

Do you find that the harder you try, the "behinder" you get? It is because there's an interference in your journey from all kinds of things—circumstances, thoughts, and temptations. The apostle Paul identified with you. As an apostle, he had his own journey of overcoming. He shared it with us when he confessed that sometimes he did the very things he didn't want to do.

In Romans, chapter 7, Paul was saying, in essence, "If I practice unforgiveness, it overtakes me. I hate it. I know I should always forgive, but for some reason, I find myself holding grudges and records of wrongs and practicing unforgiveness. When I hate unforgiveness but can't stop myself from practicing unforgiveness, it is the same as saying that the law of God—the law of forgiveness—is evil and the law of unforgiveness is good."

For that which I do I allow not: for what I would, that do I not; but what I hate, that do I. If then I do that which I would not, I consent unto the law that it is good. Now then it is no more I that do it, but sin that dwelleth in me.   (Romans 7:15–17)

Do you know that when you practice the law of sin after you know the law of God, you're calling God's Word evil and Satan's word good through your actions? I hope you really understand me. I don't mean to distress you with truth, but you need to really think about what I just said. I want you to win this war and be free from the diseases that can come upon you, but there are rules of the road, folks.

So, these two laws are battling inside you. As you will see in our investigation of spiritual roots, the law of God brings health. The law of sin brings disease. The question for you to consider is this: Which law are you being influenced by today?

THE LINK BETWEEN DISOBEDIENCE AND DISEASE

I began this journey of discovery about disobedience and disease over thirty years ago. At the beginning of my ministry, I was asked to pastor a small church. We believed in the biblical power of prayer for healing. James 5:14–15 says, "*Is any sick among you? let him call for the elders of the church; and let them pray over him, anointing him with oil in the name of the Lord: and the prayer of faith shall save the sick, and the Lord shall raise him up; and if he have committed sins, they shall be forgiven him.*"

During my first six months representing God, about 95 percent of the people who were prayed for were healed. But then things came to a screeching halt. The numbers were reversed, and less than 5 percent of those who came for prayer were healed in the following months. After incurring a 95-percent failure, I thought it was time to talk to God. I didn't have the heart to represent Scriptures from God when it wasn't working.

How would you feel if you prayed for somebody who didn't get well? It was a horrible feeling. I don't know any pastor, leader, or head of a ministry who knows what to do next when prayer doesn't work. They just don't know what to do. They come up with all kinds of reasons why it isn't working, such as, "You didn't have enough faith," "God doesn't heal today," and on and on. The list becomes longer and longer. As a young pastor, I entered into that wasteland.

One day, I went to God and said, "Sir, why is it that You honored my prayers for a short time, but now there's not much happening? Am I in gross sin? Have You released me from my assignment? Because, Sir, I'm gonna be honest with You: I don't really have the heart to pray and minister to people and have nothing happen. How can I represent You if nothing happens? Why aren't You healing these people?"

In my mind, God replied, "Henry, if you are representing Me, and you pray for someone and I don't heal them, there's a reason. I'm not their Lord." The next thing God said shook me to my core. Now, understand that these were words that were forming in my mind. God said, "Henry, Satan can have a legal right to My people's lives." (I want to restate here that not all disease comes to people in this way, and I do not believe that every single disease has a spiritual root of sin. But I have found that, without question, 80 percent of the chronic diseases that we confront have a spiritual root.)

"How can this be God speaking to me?" I wondered. I had learned that when you were saved, the curse was broken, Satan's kingdom was defeated, and you got to go free. But God said, "Yes, that did happen at the cross, but many of My people are trying to live in disobedience over something that was paid for in obedience. That's when I'm not their Lord. Jesus was obedient to Me, Henry, even to death. My people aren't."

"Well, what am I going to do with that?" I asked Him. "If You're saying that the devil has a legal right to Your people's lives in spite of what Jesus did on the cross, I need to see that in Scripture, please." That is called an honest conversation with God.

The Lord led me to 2 Timothy 2:24–26:

And the servant of the Lord must not strive; but be gentle unto all men, apt to teach, patient, in meekness instructing those that oppose themselves; if God peradventure will give them repentance to the acknowledging of the truth; and that they may recover themselves out of the snare of the devil, who are taken captive by him at his will.

(2 Timothy 2:24–26)

Whoa, what? *"Recover themselves out of the snare of the devil"?* *"Who are taken captive by him at his will"?* "Sir," I prayed, "this letter is written to Christians; how can this be happening?"

THE SNARE OF THE ENEMY

My eyes were opened when I realized what Paul was saying in this passage from 2 Timothy. His words reveal that there can be something in a Christian's life that gives the devil a legal right to steal their blessings and put a curse of disease on them. Jesus linked the law of sin to disease more than once in the New Testament. In the gospel of John, He meets the paralyzed man lying beside the pool of Bethesda. Jesus heals the man by telling him to take up his bed and walk. Hours later, Jesus is telling that same man that now that he is healed, he should go and sin no more, or something much worse will happen to him:

Jesus saith unto him, Rise, take up thy bed, and walk. And immediately the man was made whole, and took up his bed, and walked: and on the same day was the sabbath....Afterward Jesus findeth him in the temple, and said unto him, Behold, thou art made whole: sin no more, lest a worse thing come unto thee. (John 5:8–9, 14)

Disease had come to this man through the law of sin, and Jesus encouraged him by saying he had been made whole. He was not just physically well, but his sins were also forgiven, and that led to the healing of his body. At other times, when Jesus healed someone, He used the phrases "you are healed" and "your sins are forgiven" together. This is a significant connection that should not be overlooked. By joining them together, Jesus is indicating that our sins' being forgiven and our bodies' being healed have a cause-and-effect relationship. The blessing of healing coming to our physical body is the result of sin being cleansed from our spirit by forgiveness.

And, behold, they brought to him a man sick of the palsy, lying on a bed: and Jesus seeing their faith said unto the sick of the palsy; Son, be of good cheer; thy sins be forgiven thee. And, behold, certain of the scribes said within themselves, This man blasphemeth. And Jesus knowing their thoughts said, Wherefore think ye evil in your hearts? For whether is easier, to say, Thy sins be forgiven thee; or to say, Arise, and walk? But that ye may know that the Son of man hath power on earth to forgive sins, (then saith he to the sick of the palsy,) Arise, take up thy bed, and go unto thine house. (Matthew 9:2–6)

The simple fact is this: there are sicknesses that are the result of our accepting the law of sin into our lives.

THE POWER OF GRACE AND MERCY

I don't want anyone to be discouraged about the battle we face between the law of sin and the law of God. God is showing us truth for freedom's sake! When Paul looked at the truth of the battle in his own life, he cried out, "Who will save me?" Then, he answered his own question. "*O wretched man that I am! who shall deliver me from the body of this death? I thank God through Jesus Christ our Lord. So then with the mind I myself serve the law of God; but with the flesh the law of sin*" (Romans 7:24–25).

Jesus's life, death, and resurrection brought us the Father's grace and mercy. We are still living in that dispensation today. God's grace gives us the power to make the right choice. A true biblical definition of the word *grace* in the New Testament Greek is found in *Strong's Concordance.* It is "divine influence upon the [human] heart, and [the heart's] reflection in the life." Grace is God teaching you what you need to know as a child of God. Grace is God teaching you that the Holy Spirit will give you the power to defeat the influence of Satan and the law of sin in your life.

Grace's companion is mercy. *Mercy* can be defined as "the amount of time God gives us to figure out what He is saying to us through His Word and through His Spirit."

Mercy is an important New Testament concept. Under the law of Moses, certain sins required stoning or death. One example that required stoning under the Old Testament law is found in the New Testament account of the young Corinthian man who was fornicating with his father's wife. Instead of being put to death, this man was put out of the church so that he could repent to Father God and not remain under the curse of sin. He was given mercy, or a measure of time, to figure out what God had said instead of being put to death. For some people who take a long time to figure out what God is saying to them, His mercy extends exponentially. That's what His grace and mercy are all about. Aren't you glad that we are living in the dispensation of both grace and mercy?

RESPONDING TO GOD IN LOVE

Through Jesus Christ, Father God has removed the power of the law of sin and given us the opportunity for our conscience to respond to Him. Rather than responding to avoid death, we may now respond to God because we love Him and want to live in Him. We now understand that if we find sin in our hearts, we can repent and turn from it, and allow our heavenly Father to renew us in His grace and mercy.

It's a daily journey, isn't it? Through Jesus's sacrificial obedience at the cross, the devil was defeated. And by the power of the Holy Spirit, by whom Jesus was resurrected from the dead, we have a Comforter who resides with us, teaching us how to overcome Satan's kingdom day by day.

And I will pray the Father, and he shall give you another Comforter, that he may abide with you for ever; even the Spirit of truth; whom the world cannot receive, because it seeth him not, neither knoweth him: but ye know him; for he dwelleth with you, and shall be in you.

(John 14:16–17)

The plain truth is that Satan's kingdom wants you to believe God is responsible for sin and responsible for disease. If Satan can keep you confused about the source of sickness and convince you that there are no curses or consequences for sin, you can never be free. There are literally thousands of people who have come through For My Life who were told by the medical community that there was no hope for them. They were given a death sentence of disease, and they turned to God instead. When they grabbed hold of the truth of God's Word and repented of having believed Satan's lies, they had a second chance at life.

So, what is the truth? God does not want to kill you through disease! He wants you saved and restored! He hates sin, but He does not hate you! You are not sin, and once you repent of sin you can be freed and healed.

As we continue this journey together, we will be dispelling myths and superstitions that have crept into Christianity. There are many wonderful parts of the Bible that have been mishandled and misapplied because of people's desperation to be healed and blessed, and I intend to challenge them—for your freedom. It is important to settle our hearts that indeed only *good* gifts come from the Father of lights—Father God. He is not fickle, and He does not change His opinion about us from day to day. His Word is for our edification and freedom, not our cursing and disease.

Do not err, my beloved brethren. Every good gift and every perfect gift is from above, and cometh down from the Father of lights, with whom is no variableness, neither shadow of turning. Of his own will begat he us with the word of truth, that we should be a kind of firstfruits of his creatures. (James 1:16–18)

THREE

THE BIBLICAL ROLE OF PRAYER IN HEALING

I was disheartened in my early ministry when God was not answering all of my prayers for people's healing.

As I began to investigate debilitating illnesses such as Multiple Chemical Sensitivity/Environmental Illness (MCS/EI), I was forced to search the Word for any direction God might have on healing in addition to prayer. People were struggling with many allergies and sensitivities that were life-threatening. It became clear that their chemical imbalances and compromised immune responses were directly related to living stressed out and fearful lives. In order for their bodies to respond in a healthy way, they needed a change of spirituality to come back to peace—they needed repentance for believing the lies of the spirit of fear.

For My Life retreats were born out of the desire to help these and many other sick people find the spiritual change they needed for healing. Through the ministry, it is true that we have seen people healed through prayer, but we have also seen people healed when they repented to Father God without prayer. After years of these experiences, we have a very different perspective on prayer and healing from much of Christianity.

As I have held Be in Health conferences around the world in hotels, ministry centers, and churches, I found that prayer is often the exclusive means of dealing with disease and physical problems in much of the church.

There is no "plan B" if it doesn't produce healing. The elders lay hands on a person according to the words found in James, chapter 5, as the sole means of hope for healing.

Is any sick among you? let him call for the elders of the church; and let them pray over him, anointing him with oil in the name of the Lord: and the prayer of faith shall save the sick, and the Lord shall raise him up; and if he have committed sins, they shall be forgiven him.

(James 5:14–15)

Now, I am not saying there is anything wrong with laying hands on people to be healed. It is in God's Word. We do the same. However, have you ever considered the rest of this verse in James? It says, "*...if he have committed sins, they shall be forgiven him.*" Is it possible the church is only addressing part of the problem when they pray for healing? Perhaps prayer needs to be recontextualized as part of the overall picture of healing and health.

Please understand, I have experienced a great deal of opposition in my lifetime because of exposing the spiritual roots of disease. It is because I recognize that the conditions of 80 percent of people with chronic illness are directly related to the way they think, speak, and act. With my observations from science, medicine, and the Bible, my position seems uncontroversial to me, but many Christians are highly offended by this insight. Why?

Because many Christians do not want to believe they need to "repent." In the church and even in the world, the word *repent* is only used to convict "evil people" of sin to turn from their wicked ways. The truth is we all have sinned—believers and unbelievers alike. To presume otherwise is to live in denial. "*For all have sinned, and come short of the glory of God*" (Romans 3:23).

There are just as many nonbelievers as Christians who attend the For My Life retreats. As we like to say, "We don't check your 'born-again' card at the door." And it's true. The problems with humans are universal because everyone has sin in their life. Unfortunately, it offends many people to suggest that the way they think, speak, and act has caused them to become sick. They would rather believe it was just an unfortunate coincidence—a problem due to happenstance. Perhaps the reason many pastors do not address this issue is because they are afraid they might offend someone, but I believe it is worth the risk of offending you if it leads to your freedom and healing. Wouldn't you agree?

REPENTANCE AND HEALING

Nearly twenty years ago, *Newsweek* magazine featured an article that startled the scientific community. Research was uncovered that forgiveness and unforgiveness affect human health.[5] When medical science made this discovery, some people declared that unforgiveness is a disease because they recognized its effect on the human body. However, that's not what the Bible calls it. The Bible calls unforgiveness a sin. Our biggest problem is that people want to be healed without getting rid of the sins that are at the root of the disease. Forgiveness has to come first. Don't hold on to the wrongs committed by others. Be a doer of the Word. Be a forgiver.

In order to prove my point, I want to begin by sharing a story of hope. This is the account of someone who was miraculously healed from a life-threatening disease through the power of repentance from unforgiveness.

Several years ago, I had the opportunity to minister to a pastor's wife who was diagnosed with stage IV breast cancer. It had metastasized, so she was given no hope for survival. She'd been prayed for by her husband and the elders of their church, but there was no change. Her doctor, who attended their church, heard about my work with disease, especially healing from cancer, and told her, "Maybe you should call Pastor Wright; he's your last resort."

One afternoon, I received a call from the woman's husband. He shared that she'd been referred to me by her doctor and that she was dying of cancer. A minute later, the wife got on the phone and quietly asked me, "Dr.

---

5. Jerry Adler, "Forgive and Let Live," *Newsweek*, October 3, 2004, https://www.newsweek.com/forgive-and-let-live-129513.

Wright, will you pray for me?" Sincere Christians had already prayed for her many times. Had she been healed? No. If I had just prayed for her, she would be dead by now. This is when it's vital to know the Word of God. There are times when we just don't understand it like we need to.

"No, I'm not going to pray for you," I answered her.

Shocked, she replied, "But you're supposed to. Why did my doctor send me to you if you're not going to pray for me?"

Well, I suppose that was a legitimate question. I replied, "No, I don't have to pray for you; I have to follow the Word."

She said, "Follow the Word? The Word says you're supposed to pray for me. Why won't you pray for me?"

"Because you have committed a sin that is unto death," I answered truthfully, "and the Word says that if I see my brother or my sister commit a sin that is unto death, I should not pray for it." I was referring to 1 John 5:16–17, which says, "*If any man see his brother sin a sin which is not unto death, he shall ask, and he shall give him life for them that sin not unto death. There is a sin unto death: I do not say that he shall pray for it. All unrighteousness is sin: and there is a sin not unto death.*"

UNFORGIVENESS IS A SIN

Before I continue the testimony, I want you to think about this. If all unrighteousness is sin, do you think that unforgiveness is righteousness or unrighteousness? It is unrighteousness, and therefore it is sin. So, if you followed unforgiveness, you would be following the law of sin. Are you tracking with me? The person who has been nurturing unforgiveness is following the law of sin, which has produced a disease that is "unto death." When I say it is "unto death," I mean that healing can be blocked if the root spiritual issue that led to the deadly physical disease is not dealt with. If it is not addressed, the natural course of the disease will cause the person's death. It's a spiritual root, and it has to be dealt with before healing can take place.

I read this Scripture in 1 John 5:16–17 to the pastor's wife who was dying of cancer, and she asked me, "Well, what is my sin?" That was also a legitimate question, but I wouldn't tell her. Why? Because I didn't want her to give me the "right answer" just because of her fear of dying. I wanted the conviction to come from within her, from her own heart. I didn't want to coach her. It's easy to say yes to somebody coaching you. It's another thing to search your own heart for the truth.

Although I wouldn't tell her, I knew from my three-decade journey of fighting disease that a high percentage of case histories reveal that a woman who gets breast cancer is someone who has bitterness and unforgiveness in her life. In over 80 percent of those cases, that unforgiveness is against another woman.

Finally, I said, "Let me ask you a question. Do you have any unforgiveness or bitterness against another woman?" She became really quiet. After some time, she admitted, "Yes, I do." I started to get excited inside, but I didn't want it to show. Why was I so excited? Because in James 5:16, it says, *"Confess your faults one to another, and pray one for another, that ye may be healed."* I knew that her healing required confession.

WE MUST BE HONEST WITH OURSELVES

I want to be clear here. If she had said no, the call would have been finished, and she'd probably be dead today. But she admitted to harboring unforgiveness, so I responded, "Good. Thank you for your honesty. What do you think you should do next?"

"I think I should call the unforgiveness sin."

"Okay," I answered. "That's good. What do you think you need to do with that sin that you've been practicing against this woman?"

"Well, I think I need to go to the Father and ask Him to forgive me."

Now, if I had said, "Good. Do it!" and ended it there, she would still have been in trouble. There was more to it.

Forgiving others is one of the major keys to receiving from God. When this woman said, "I think I need to repent to the Father," I said, "Very good." I was getting more excited, but I wouldn't let her know. I asked her, "What else do you need to do?" because I was hearing two Scripture verses in my mind. Jesus said, in Matthew 6:15, *"But if ye forgive not men their trespasses, neither will your Father forgive your trespasses."* And in Mark 11:26,

He said, "*But if ye do not forgive, neither will your Father which is in heaven forgive your trespasses.*

She thought for a minute and then said, "Well, I think what I need to do is not just confess to the Father. I need to contact this woman, confess to her that I've had this bitterness, and ask her to forgive me."

TAKE RESPONSIBILITY FOR YOUR LIFE

The pastor's wife made the life-changing decision to take responsibility for her bitterness against this other woman by forgiving her and asking for her forgiveness. She decided to get in contact with her and say, "I've had this bitterness. I hate it. It is sin in my life. I ask you to forgive me." I knew that when she confessed to the Father and asked for forgiveness from the woman, she would be forgiven. I knew the power of the cross would work in her life. It doesn't matter that it was metastasized cancer—the power of the enemy was broken over her. Nothing could hinder her healing. If she took care of that unforgiveness with a pure heart of conviction, nothing would keep her from God at any level.

Once she told me she was going to repent to the Father and contact the woman, I said, "I'm so glad you called me."

"Are you going to pray for me now?" she asked.

"I don't have to," I replied. "If you're sincerely repentant, you have met the conditions of the cross, and the power of death is defeated in your life. Go your way and sin no more."

Well, I never heard from her again. But, a few months later, I received a book in the mail entitled *The Biblical Guide to Alternative Medicine*, autographed by the author, Dr. Michael Jacobson. He was the woman's medical doctor who attended their church in Cincinnati and had counseled her to call me.

One of the chapters in his book is dedicated to what science calls mind-body medicine. (We will cover this subject in more detail later.) When I read this chapter, I discovered that the pastor's wife had received a complete healing from her cancer! In the case study, Dr. Jacobson referenced "a pastor from Georgia" who had ministered in the healing of this woman. Even though I wasn't mentioned by name, I was happy to hear that the cancer had disappeared structure-wide, and that God had also healed all the damage previously done to her body by the disease. This woman remains cancer free today. God was faithful to His Word.

How did her healing occur? She had to be obedient. Her heart was open and submitted to the Word. She confessed and repented of her sin, first to Father God and then to the person against whom she had been harboring bitterness. She became a doer of the Word and not just a hearer, which the Bible warns against: *"But be ye doers of the word, and not hearers only, deceiving your own selves"* (James 1:22).

Why was it important that she become a doer of the Word? So that she would no longer deceive herself, and she could recover herself from "the snare of the devil"! *"And that they may recover themselves out of the snare of the devil, who are taken captive by him at his will"* (2 Timothy 2:26).

I get really excited about the truth of God's Word. People will say to me, "You need to calm down, Henry." Why would they want me to calm down? It's amazing how many people take issue with the passion I have about the calling on my life. But I am my brother's keeper. The blood of my brother is crying out from the church, demanding justice, demanding the truth on the healing of disease. My role is giving people knowledge so that they can *"recover themselves out of the snare of the devil,"* just as it says in God's Word. I want to help you recover yourself from the snare of the devil.

Paul shared the above verse with us because we need to know the truth in order to be brought to repentance. Repentance is not a bad word. Having to repent doesn't mean that you are not a Christian or that you are an evil person. Paul was speaking to New Testament believers when he talked about repentance.

PRAYER, REPENTANCE, AND SANCTIFICATION

I want you to reconsider the role of prayer especially as it relates to repentance. If you are going to have meaningful, long-lasting relationships, I believe you are going to have to do two things to be successful: communicate and repent. This includes with Father God. We should not be scared of going to the Father of all spirits, the Lord of creation, and saying, "Father,

I'm sorry. I come to You in Jesus's name. Father, I've yielded to Satan's law of sin. I've been following it, but I've hated it. I don't want to do it anymore. As it says in Your Word, it's not good for me. I come to You to take responsibility, and I repent to You for allowing the law of sin to control my life. Will You please forgive me?"

Is that hard? There's no copay when you get that kind of prescription. No insurance is needed. Yet it may save you from incurable diseases. You can do a lot to prevent disease in your life when you communicate openly with Father God, admitting when you have fallen into sin. It is not time to hide from Him but to be transparent when you have missed the mark.

Prayers of repentance and sanctification play important roles in disease prevention or becoming free from disease. That's why we are going to consider both of them. We're so busy chasing symptoms and disease profiles that we don't even take into account why we got sick to begin with. Oftentimes, we need to deal with sin and spiritual issues that are affecting our hearts before our healing can occur.

We experience *repentance* from our sins when we first turn to God to acknowledge Jesus Christ's death and resurrection on our behalf. That is our salvation. As Christians, we still need further repentance for things in our lives that aren't of God. We need to allow God to continually change us. That is our *sanctification*. Sanctification is a lifelong process for Christians whereby, through the glories and trials of life, and through our obedience to God, we learn to *"walk in newness of life"*: *"That like as Christ was raised up from the dead by the glory of the Father, even so we also should walk in newness of life"* (Romans 6:4).

It would be great if, once we became Christians, we never sinned again, yet that isn't so. The book of 1 John tells us that Christians still sin, but that God is always gracious to forgive our sins.

If we say that we have no sin, we deceive ourselves, and the truth is not in us. If we confess our sins, he is faithful and just to forgive us our sins, and to cleanse us from all unrighteousness. If we say that we have not sinned, we make him a liar, and his word is not in us.

(1 John 1:8–10)

IT'S CONVICTION, NOT CONDEMNATION!

Now, it's important that you don't react to God's truth about sin in your life by feeling condemned and running away from your Bible. The Holy Spirit convicts us of sin so that we might be brought to repentance and freedom, not condemnation. The Holy Spirit's conviction helps us to recognize our sin so that we can repent of it and walk in the freedom of Jesus Christ. It says in Romans 8:1, *"There is therefore now no condemnation to them which are in Christ Jesus, who walk not after the flesh, but after the Spirit."*

Sanctification does not represent the removal of your free will and personality. Father God does not want you to become a robot. Instead, sanctification represents the removal of the sin that brings torment and separation from God. He desires you to follow Him and be transformed, but He will not force you to do so. God reveals sanctification to us in several places in Scripture. For example, we read in 2 Corinthians 3:18, *"But we all, with open face beholding as in a glass the glory of the Lord, are changed into the same image from glory to glory, even as by the Spirit of the Lord."*

The words *"are changed into the same image"* are in the progressive present tense. That means that being changed into Christ's image is an ongoing process. We are learning to follow after Christ day by day. When people ask how I'm doing, I reply, "I'm walking in a straight wavy line." What does that mean? It means I desire to follow God in a straight line, but the reality of my journey is that I seem pretty wavy at times. Do I know how to follow God "perfectly"? Of course not. I make mistakes, and the Holy Spirit convicts me of sin so that I may repent.

Remember that 1 Thessalonians 5:23 states, *"The very God of peace sanctify you wholly"*—reminding us that we would be made blameless in spirit, soul, and body until the coming of the Lord Jesus Christ? Well, Jesus hasn't come back yet. So, guess what we're doing? We are still being sanctified in our spirits, sanctified in our souls, and sanctified in our bodies. Our minds are being renewed: *"And be not conformed to this world: but be ye transformed by the renewing of your mind"* (Romans 1:2). We are being changed spiritually. As a result, our bodies are going to sing and rejoice and leap for joy! We will be in health!

That is God's plan for us. Our part is to embrace His truth, repent of following any aspect of the law of sin, and allow Him to transform us into His image. We are saved by God's forgiveness and mercy, but we walk out our sanctification on a daily basis. That is why God gives us the responsibility of believing the truth of the Word when it comes to our health and healing.

Now, God is not going to live your life for you! You have to take ownership in this victory. You have the choice to follow Father God or to follow after sin. I implore you to wake up! I'm in your corner, rooting for you to make a quality decision to repent to Father God of your sin. You must decide to be an overcomer, to face the challenges of life and defeat them, in Jesus's name.

LET GOD SEARCH YOUR HEART

When people become angry or challenge me over these teachings, they talk about legalism and scare tactics. They accuse me of saying that all disease is spiritually rooted. Again, I have said I believe 80 percent of incurable diseases are spiritually rooted. Therefore, I also believe there are 20 percent that are not. However, if you have a disease that we consider to be in that 80 percent, wouldn't you want to search the Scriptures to find out why you are sick? It is crucial to pray and ask God for the reason why you are sick and trust He will show you in His Word. We should do more than petition Father God for healing when we are sick; we should also pray and ask Him to reveal our hearts to us.

King David understood this as he asked God to search his heart, saying, *"Search me, O God, and know my heart: try me, and know my thoughts: and see if there be any wicked way in me, and lead me in the way everlasting"* (Psalm 139:23–24).

If what is keeping you from your healing is choosing the law of sin—which is the opposite of the Word of God—wouldn't you want to be convicted of it, confess it, and move on to a life of wholeness and health? I know that I would, and I have. I pray that as you learn these truths, the Father, in Jesus's name, will release the Holy Spirit to give you a hunger to search the Scriptures more and more. In God's Word, you have a lamp for the journey of life. Psalm 119:105 says, *"Thy word is a lamp unto my feet, and a light unto my path."*

REFLECTING GOD'S NATURE OR SATAN'S?

Why do we talk to one another and communicate with one another? These practices build trust so we can work with one another and care for one another. This is foundational to a proper relationship with other humans. The same is also true in our relationship with Father God. If we wish to get to know Him, we need to talk to Him (pray), we need to listen to Him (read the Bible), and we need to apply His instructions. As we learn to do this, we will reflect His nature as part of our nature. This is an essential fruit of sanctification.

However, what happens when we do the opposite and listen to Satan's kingdom instead? Is it possible we will become a reflection of the enemy's kingdom if we apply our hearts to what the enemy has said?

The sin of bitterness is one major area where we can become a reflection of Satan's kingdom. When we minister to individuals at For My Life, we can tell when they are bitter because of one phrase: "So-and-so hurt me." If a person uses this one statement, we recognize they have unforgiveness in their life. When we are wronged by someone, we have a decision to make in that moment. I believe that "we are called to be 'pierced' but not wounded." What does that mean? It means we are not robots. If someone says or does something evil to us, we may feel "pierced," and we may feel "hurt." However, what we do afterward is the difference between sin and temptation. If we choose to release the offense to Father God and forgive the individual, then we will remain free from bitterness. However, if we embrace the offense and choose to hold on to the "hurt," we will take in that offense as a sort of spiritual "wound." It will continue to trouble us unless we finally repent to Father God and forgive the person who hurt us.

When you take on an offense and choose not to forgive, you become a "god" in the situation with the goal of judging right from wrong for yourself. You decide whether to get revenge or to protect yourself. Bitterness is an ugly sin that corrodes like acid, eating away at your soul. First, it poisons the mind, and then it poisons the body.

There are worsening degrees of bitterness that develop once the root of unforgiveness has taken hold. Bitterness begins with unforgiveness and then moves to resentment, retaliation, anger/wrath, hatred, violence, and finally murder, even if it is not the physical murder of the person you are bitter toward but murder with the tongue. I have found without exception that if someone has one of the more advanced degrees of bitterness, the other degrees of bitterness are sure to be a part of the person's life.

For instance, if a person is angry, I can predict that they also struggle with retaliation, resentment, and unforgiveness. And we have this warning in Hebrews 12:15: *"Looking diligently lest any man fail of the grace of God; lest any root of bitterness springing up trouble you, and thereby many be defiled."*

CANCER AND BITTERNESS

To expand on the earlier testimony of the pastor's wife, I want to share the full insight we have come to understand around the spiritual roots of breast cancer. Through thirty-plus years of confronting cancer, we have seen proven statistics and many testimonies of healing. Now, I know that there are always exceptions, but we have seen the following results in a high percentage of testimonies and case histories over the years.

If a woman comes for healing from breast cancer in the right breast, in our experience, her unforgiveness is toward a non-blood relative. So, the first thing I ask her is, "Are you married?" If she answers, "Yes," I further ask, "What is your relationship with your mother-in-law?" Most of the time, it's not very good, because I have found that, statistically, the number one cause of breast cancer in the right breast is unresolved bitterness and unforgiveness between a woman and her mother-in-law. If you have ears to hear, ladies, make sure you're okay with your mother-in-law.

I had a man come to our ministry office a few years ago whose wife had cancer in her right breast. I had them both in my office, and I asked her, "How are you with your mother-in-law?" Her husband was sitting right there. She huffed up and said, "We were pretty good until she came to live with us!" "Then what?" I asked. "He built her a nice apartment over the garage." "Okay, what's wrong with that?" "We can be sitting down at dinner, and his mother calls for him, which is often. He'll leave me and let the dinner go cold to attend to her. I think he's married to his mother!" Do you think she had some bitterness? Even if you're not in ministry and don't have the experience, you already know the answer.

If the cancer appears in a woman's left breast over the heart, statistically, it is related to unresolved bitterness in the woman with another female who is a blood relative. At the top of the list is a biological mother or biological sister. It's held true enough times that I am confident to make it a statistical observation.

I have seen these cancers disappear as a result of sincere repentance and forgiveness. After decades of ministering on disease, I have enough confidence to tell you that 80 percent of cases of breast cancer, whether in the right or the left breast, are not due to happenstance. It is the work of the enemy because unforgiveness and bitterness is the law of sin, and you are not to have bitterness against anyone.

TAKING IN ANOTHER PERSON'S SIN?

When you decide to follow the law of sin and hold a record of wrongs against another person, it will very likely produce a disease in your body. That's true even when that person truly sinned against you. They opened their mouth and said something or did something that wronged you. They betrayed you. They destroyed something precious to you. Yes, they did it. It was their sin. But because of your agreement with a spirit of bitterness, you now have a disease.

I need to ask you a very serious question. I don't want you to ever forget this question for as long as you live, because your life depends on it.

Why would you take the sins of another person into your body?

What do I mean by "take the sins of another person into your body"? When you choose to harbor bitterness and to stew on an offence, it may eventually produce diseases such as cancer in your body. That person may have wronged you, but now you may face the consequences in your spirit and your body for not forgiving them. It doesn't harm them. It harms you! Jesus paid the price for that sin. He went to the cross and shed His blood for the forgiveness of sins, including your sins and the sins of the person who offended you. Why would you die of disease for the sin of another against you?

We need a paradigm shift. If our perspective is simply to resist bitterness when people offend us, that is not a completed work. When people look at us, are they just going to see a "non-bitter" person? No. They need to be able to see a loving person. You need to make an important decision. Are you willing to forgive despite any wrong done to you?

But love ye your enemies, and do good, and lend, hoping for nothing again; and your reward shall be great, and ye shall be the children of the Highest: for he is kind unto the unthankful and to the evil. Be ye therefore merciful, as your Father also is merciful. Judge not, and ye shall not be judged: condemn not, and ye shall not be condemned: forgive, and ye shall be forgiven. (Luke 6:35–37)

How do you live out this command to forgive your enemies? The first step is to understand what forgiveness is and what it is not. It is not making sin "okay." Some people believe that forgiveness is rationalizing sin committed against us. Such individuals are tormented because they have been severely abused and cannot see a way of being fine with what was done to them. The good news is you do not need to call sin good. Sin is evil.

The next important decision you need to make is to release the person and their sin against you to Father God. The truth of the matter is that every single human will have to give an account to God for their life and their decisions after they die. No one gets away with anything. If someone means you harm, they are living with the same torment they are manifesting toward you. Remember, it is out of the abundance of the heart that both good and evil come. It is not those things that we eat that defile us, but the things we do and say that defile us and make us feel ashamed and guilty.

O generation of vipers, how can ye, being evil, speak good things? for out of the abundance of the heart the mouth speaketh. A good man out of the good treasure of the heart bringeth forth good things: and an evil man out of the evil treasure bringeth forth evil things. But I say unto you, That every idle word that men shall speak, they shall give account thereof in the day of judgment.   (Matthew 12:34–36)

Your decision requires releasing others and their sins against you to Father God with the understanding that He will take care of you and take care of them. Forgiveness requires relinquishing control to Father God and not being your own defender.

THE CANCER PROFILE

Our decades of experience at Be in Health have led to some important observations about many individuals struggling with cancer in general.

The following are characteristics we have found:

1. A tendency to respond to anger and stress with hopelessness and despair to the point of being shut down

2. A marked inability to forgive

3. A tendency toward self-pity and self-introspection

4. A poor ability to develop and maintain meaningful long-term relationships without fear

5. A great tendency to hold resentment

6. Poor self-image

7. The loss of a serious love object up to 24 months prior to the cancer, or the continued grief and unresolved issues relative to the love object

8. The loss of a significant life role or purpose in life

9. Being fired or rejected in a vocational or avocational pursuit

10. Loss of hope

11. Hope deferred

12. Denial about personal feelings and needs

These characteristics are not meant to bring discouragement if you have been diagnosed with cancer. However, if any part of this list fits your life experience, then hopefully we can shine a light on what these characteristics represent and how Father God can restore your life and your health.

The overarching thread that ties together the experiences and tendencies on this list is a lack of hope and love in a person's life. The key is found in the first point. When a person is unable to deal with stress and anger by addressing challenges in their life in a healthy way, the general result is to "shut down." By "shut down," I mean exactly what it sounds like. This person is unable to address conflict or disappointment without turning inward or avoiding the problem altogether. They shut down the situation and "stuff" their emotions inside, often pretending certain problems do not trouble them at all. However, the truth is that these situations are eating them up on the inside.

Since temptation from Satan's kingdom comes in the form of negative thoughts, feelings, and emotions, the only way we can resist becoming bitter and angry when we feel offended is to grab hold of the truth. The Word of God does not say we are to be led by our emotions and feelings. Instead, we must make the choice to be led by the Word of God despite what we feel.

LIFE IS NOT A FORMULA

The reality is that sometimes in life there are unfortunate or painful situations that cannot be remedied easily. The loss of a loved one or a purpose or role in life is one example. Other individuals have hopes that have never come to pass or that have been "deferred." Perhaps a woman is past her childbearing years and has always believed that if *only* she could have been a mother, then her life would have been happy and fulfilled. In other circumstances, people have built their career around their accomplishments, and once they retire or have their reputation marred by false accusations or being fired, they lose their hope. A sense of hopelessness and depression may take hold.

Ironically, the core problem often lies with the hope that has been deferred. It is easy for our expectations and hopes—to have a successful career, to be married, to have children—to become idols. It is not evil to have hopes and desires, but our ultimate hope must be in the Lord. Even if we lose everything we have, we must be willing to entrust our life to Father God and release our hopes to Him. It may seem daunting because we have centered our life on these hopes, but these same desires going unfulfilled or dominating our thoughts may, in fact, be killing us.

Life is not a formula. There is not a series of steps for avoiding the hard parts. However, there are important keys from Scripture that give us a route to faith and hope. Our hope cannot be based upon what we can see and what we can control. Faith is not the substance of what we can see. Faith is the substance of what we *cannot* see. As the Bible describes it, *"Now faith is the substance of things hoped for, the evidence of things not seen"* (Hebrews 11:1). God's Word commends faith, saying, *"Blessed is the man that trusteth in the LORD, and whose hope the LORD is"* (Jeremiah 17:7).

PRAYER IS ABOUT MORE THAN HEALING!

We began this chapter addressing the purpose of prayer in healing. On a basic level, I define prayer in a simple way: talking to God. Sadly, many people believe prayer is a religious duty only to be performed in certain situations. Too often, we remove the simplicity of prayer, which is open communication and conversation with our Father God who loves us. When Christians only see Father God as someone who is there to meet their own needs, those needs occupy the bulk of their prayer time. We must get our eyes off of ourselves. The world is filled with people who are hurting and alone. They do not know God, and they do not know how to love and care for one another.

Remember, disease is a result of separation, including from other humans. Instead of focusing primarily on healing for our physical bodies, maybe our prayer life needs to focus on being part of the spiritual solution and not the spiritual pollution of sin. It is time to engage with Father God and ask Him to teach us how to love a world that may not love us. We need to ask Him to show us how to forgive and reengage even with those people who may have done harm to us in the past. We must trust Him to give us wisdom for how closely we will associate with them based upon the conviction of the Holy Spirit in our lives. There may be those who are too caustic to be around, but the question is, are you willing to love them and pray for the restoration of relationship even at a distance?

I believe God will teach us how to pray for others and how to trust Him every day. I want to leave you with the prayer model Jesus gave to His disciples, commonly called the Lord's Prayer, as a reminder of what Father God sees as important for us to focus on in prayer:

And he said unto them, When ye pray, say, Our Father which art in heaven, hallowed be thy name. Thy kingdom come. Thy will be done, as in heaven, so in earth. Give us day by day our daily bread. And forgive us our sins; for we also forgive every one that is indebted to us. And lead us not into temptation; but deliver us from evil. (Luke 11:2–4)

HEALED IN TWO DAYS

TOM

Although I had always been a healthy man, I began to experience great physical distress. My bones were beginning to disintegrate from the inside out. Everything was breaking, from the bones in my feet up through my hips; even my ribs were fraying. The doctor's diagnosis was a rare condition called tumor osteomyelitis. I had an inoperable tumor that was sending a signal to my kidneys that prevented them from processing any vitamin D. I was in desperate shape; I could barely walk. I had been a Christian for years and tried to follow the Lord, but now my health was falling apart.

One day, a simple encounter changed my life. A neighbor was walking down the street while my wife was in the front yard. When the neighbor found out how ill I was, she said, "I have a book Tom needs to read." It was *A More Excellent Way* by Dr. Wright. I devoured the book in a week, and one week later, my wife and I were in Thomaston, Georgia, at a For My Life retreat.

My heart was wide open to biblical truths on health that I had never realized before. I had never understood that there were things that I needed to confess and get rid of for my health to change. After the first two days at that retreat, I went from barely being able to walk to getting rid of my crutches! I was healed!

When I returned home, I went back to my endocrinologist. Stunned, he said to me, "Tom, whatever happened to you, I didn't do it." Today, I am continuing to grow in my walk with the Lord. I have a steady confidence in my relationship with my Father. I am now able to rest and trust His love for me.

FOUR

SPIRIT-SOUL-BODY CONNECTION

Where do our thoughts come from? Is every thought we think from ourselves? More important, *how* do both God and the devil speak to us? These are vital questions we need to answer in order to understand the spiritual roots of disease. For Christians, some of our thoughts are from the Holy Spirit, and some of our thoughts are our own. But there are other thoughts that originate from the enemy.

Teaching on the spirit-soul-body connection removes much of the superstition related to the subject of how Satan's kingdom speaks to and influences humans. I have mentioned that some people become angry when I tell them that Satan can put a disease on them if they give him permission through disobedience. Believers who attend For My Life often struggle with this concept initially, even though they are suffering from diseases related to spiritual issues such as fear and bitterness. They may say, "I'm a Christian, and the Bible says I have the mind of Christ. So how is this possible?" They are referring to Paul's first letter to the Corinthians, in which he wrote, *"For who hath known the mind of the Lord, that he may instruct him? but we have the mind of Christ"* (1 Corinthians 2:16).

The problem is, what does having the mind of Christ mean? How does one have the mind of Christ? It's important to read a few additional verses in 1 Corinthians to understand this concept. First Corinthians 2:14 says, *"But the natural man receiveth not the things of the Spirit of God: for they are foolishness unto him: neither can he know them, because they are spiritually discerned."*

The natural man or unbeliever does not receive the things of the Holy Spirit, but Christians are able to do so. To have the "mind of Christ," Paul presumes in 1 Corinthians 2:16 that Christians are paying attention to what the Holy Spirit is saying to them. The truth is that the Holy Spirit is speaking to believers, but are we listening to Him? The Holy Spirit convicts humanity of sin. If Christians are struggling with the same sins and diseases as the world, perhaps we are still in need of listening to the Holy Spirit for conviction and repentance of sin. Speaking of the Holy Spirit, Jesus said, *"And when he is come, he will reprove the world of sin, and of righteousness, and of judgment"* (John 16:8).

Consider this: does your life—including your lifestyle, your decisions, and any family conflicts you may have—reflect the mind of Christ? If you truly have the mind of Christ, you know the Word, and you are a doer of the Word. We acquire the "mind of Christ" through reading our Bible, realigning our thinking with God's Word, repenting of sin, and embracing God's ways and nature. We're supposed to be moving forward in God's Word. Understanding how we are tempted is a crucial step in exposing the spiritual roots of disease. That is why we need to look at the role our mind plays in disease—this is the spirit-soul (mind)-body connection.

THE ORIGIN OF YOUR THOUGHTS

We have already acknowledged that the Holy Spirit of God is a Spirit. The enemy is a spirit. You are a spirit with a soul and a body. Your body is what interacts with the physical world, but the eternal part of you is a spirit. You cannot see your spirit with your physical eyes, but it's in you. For the believer, your body is also the temple of the Holy Spirit.

God communicates with us Spirit to spirit. Unfortunately, Satan also communicates with us spirit to spirit. We receive thoughts at the spirit level and record them at the soul (mind) level. Again, they could be our thoughts, they could come from the Holy Spirit, or they could come from the enemy. And those from the enemy bring the roots of disease with them—which can affect our body.

When a thought passes through our mind, we think it comes from us. However, it may have been given to us by an invisible enemy from an invisible kingdom who will then make it sound like it came from us by using first-person statements. The enemy might say, "I'm so angry right now," or "I'm really concerned about my life," or "I never do anything right." Satan tempts us with a thought, repeats that thought over and over, and deceives us into accepting it as our own. We embrace the thought and take ownership of it. Then, the enemy uses that thought to control us spiritually, psychologically, and biologically. Such thoughts are what the Bible calls temptations. That is why it is important for you to understand that not all of the thoughts that come to your mind are your own.

THETA BRAINWAVES AND YOUR SPIRITUALITY

From decades of research and case studies, I have drawn together an understanding of the wholeness of spirit, soul, and body from Scripture and connected it to our brainwaves. It is important to point out that my observations in this section are personal insights and not something I can substantiate entirely from scientific literature. These are personal observations we teach at For My Life to give Christians an understanding of how both the Holy Spirit and Satan's kingdom can speak to humans and influence our lives.

We all have brainwaves as a part of our cognition. Brainwaves are electrical neuropathways in the brain, each created by God with a purpose. While I recognize that we have more than three brainwaves, I want to focus on three specific ones because I intend to relate these brainwaves back to our scriptural understanding of humans—that we are a spirit, we have a soul (mind), and we live in a body.

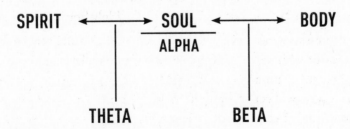

Based upon the understanding of these three separate components of our creation, I have observed three brainwaves that correspond as juncture points connecting to our spirit, soul, and body. What are these three?

The first are *beta* brainwaves. They are responsible for our waking functions related to our five physical senses. We respond and react to our world via beta brainwaves. These form a junction or connection between our *body* and our soul, or mind.

Alpha brainwaves are part of a more relaxed, thoughtful way of thinking. It is my position that this forms the specific realm of our *soul*. It is where we are creative and consider our lives, our personal decisions, and our reflective thought processes.

Of central importance to this discussion on the spirit-soul-body connection are *theta* brainwaves. Theta brainwaves form the juncture between soul and *spirit*. Theta brainwaves are the means by which both the Holy Spirit and evil spirits communicate with humans.

God wants to influence us from within by His Spirit and by His Word. He uses these theta brain waves to speak to us from within, to train us in His nature and righteousness. Unfortunately, Satan and his kingdom of darkness want to influence us from within, as well; the enemy uses theta waves, the same pathway as the Holy Spirit, to train us in the law of sin. Satan has been training the human race in the law of sin since the time of Adam and Eve. Since temptation comes to train you, be careful what you listen to, watch, and dwell on.

THE IMPORTANCE OF LONG-TERM MEMORY

At this point, there is a specific part of the spirit-soul-body connection that we need to address, and that is the concept of long-term memory. It is a biological truth that the things we think about and dwell on actually become part of who we are. We will never get to the spiritual root of disease if we don't understand the biology of how our mind affects our body.

If you meet up with someone today, your mind will take a mental picture or "snapshot" of them. Your eyes are cameras taking pictures, your ears are recorders capturing sounds; you are experiencing the world around you with your five physical senses. Your brain is taking pictures all the time, by the millions. Those pictures are electrochemical occurrences that use another electrical chemical in your brain cells to mirror the image of what you just saw, heard, tasted, smelled, or touched.

Initially, what you perceive around you is recorded in your short-term memory. In order for it to move to long-term memory, a biological event must take place in your brain called *protein synthesis*. In protein synthesis, there is a component of your genetics that plays a role in the process known as RNA. This component of RNA takes the electrochemical picture and integrates it into your brain cells permanently as a part of your long-term memory. That image, or thought, now becomes a part of you biologically, not just a mirror image stored somewhere.

Thoughts and images, whether good or evil, become permanent parts of your mind, your personality, and the way you think and act. For that reason, both God and Satan want their thoughts and images to be stored in your long-term memory. Satan will train you through long-term memory with temptations to bring on disorders and disease. God will train you through long-term memory as you meditate, or dwell, on His Word so that you can live in health and freedom. *"O how love I thy law! it is my meditation all the day"* (Psalm 119:97).

OUT OF SIGHT, OUT OF MIND?

What happens when we embrace the temptations and thoughts of the enemy instead of embracing the truth of the Word of God? That is when our minds become overwhelmed with fear, anger, self-hatred, depression, hopelessness, and much more.

Let me ask you a question. Did Jesus cast out people's emotions in the gospels? No! Jesus cast out evil spirits.

And there was in their synagogue a man with an unclean spirit; and he cried out, saying, Let us alone; what have we to do with thee, thou Jesus of Nazareth? art thou come to destroy us? I know thee who thou art, the Holy One of God. And Jesus rebuked him, saying, Hold thy peace, and come out of him. And when the unclean spirit had torn him, and cried with a loud voice, he came out of him. (Mark 1:23–26)

Many Christians do not want to address the existence of evil spirits because they are severely afraid of evil. But I need to tell you this bluntly: "Out of sight, out of mind" is *not* a spiritual principle. Perhaps many perceive the effects of an evil spirit only through the lens of the Gadarene demoniac described in the Gospels. The graphic images of horror movies and television have also trained us to be afraid of evil spirits, preventing us from learning the truth and living in freedom.

However, I believe that the biggest problem the church has with evil spirits comes from the word *possessed*. It is a term used in the King James Version of the Bible.

And his fame went throughout all Syria: and they brought unto him all sick people that were taken with divers diseases and torments, and those which were possessed with devils, and those which were lunatick, and those that had the palsy; and he healed them. (Matthew 4:24)

Many people think of the word *possessed* as being *owned* by devils. In *Strong's Concordance*, the word *possessed*, in this context, is Greek 1139. An alternate translation for it would be "vexed with." In other words, it means "troubled by." Do evil spirits trouble us? If they bring fear, unforgiveness, and bitterness, then, yes, I consider that trouble. At Be in Health, we do not believe that Christians are owned by devils. However, we do see clear evidence that they are troubled, sometimes greatly, by them.

We need to accept the truth that evil spirits do exist. Second Timothy 1:7 says that God has not given us the *spirit* of fear. Clearly, that means that the spirit of fear exists and that it can be given to vex and torment us in any area of our lives if we give it permission—and that torment can lead to disease. Many in the church explain away this Scripture as merely referring to the psychological state of being afraid, but this verse plainly states it is a *"spirit of fear"*: *"For God hath not given us the spirit of fear; but of power, and of love, and of a sound mind"* (2 Timothy 1:7).

The main argument we encounter concerning whether evil spirits can vex a Christian is based upon the belief that a Christian cannot have an evil spirit or be tempted by evil spirits. "Since the Holy Spirit comes to live with us after we are born again," they insist, "we cannot be affected or tempted by an evil spirit." The problem is, I cannot find evidence from Scripture supporting this position.

At Be in Health we have observed that indeed Christians can be greatly affected by evil spirits. Have you ever felt scattered or smothered when you have been afraid or stressed out? Have you ever found it hard to process thoughts or felt like running away when times are tough? While there is a healthy response to "fight-or-flight" situations that happen in life, there are many Christians who live an unhealthy lifestyle of being afraid on a continual basis. That is when a spirit of fear may have overtaken a part of their life.

As a believer, you were bought with a price through the sacrifice of Jesus on the cross, but that does not mean you are fully walking in the benefits of all that Jesus accomplished for you. As Paul rightly identifies, we are bought with a price, and *therefore* we should not serve sin. If believers are urged not to serve sin, doesn't that mean that sometimes we do serve sin *after* being born again?

Flee fornication. Every sin that a man doeth is without the body; but he that committeth fornication sinneth against his own body. What? know ye not that your body is the temple of the Holy Ghost which is in you, which ye have of God, and ye are not your own? For ye are bought with a price: therefore glorify God in your body, and in your spirit, which are God's. (1 Corinthians 6:18–20)

When we agree to live in sin and to embrace fear, bitterness, or unforgiveness, we are inviting evil spirits to join our life in those specific areas. At For My Life, we focus on teaching subjects from the Bible such as fear, using scriptural proofs to help attendees discern spirits of fear in their own lives. We are not generic humans, and what one person struggles with is not the same as another. One person may be afraid of failure and another person may be afraid of abuse. They both have a spirit of fear, but in different areas of their lives. Once they recognize and repent of having listened to the enemy's lies, we cast out those evil spirits so that those individuals may return to the peace of Father God.

DOES OUR PHYSICAL BODY CAUSE US TO SIN?

Another important reason we address the spirit-soul-body connection via theta brainwave activity is to respond to a core theological problem proposed by some in the church. Their claim is that evil spirits cannot tempt believers, and that the term *flesh* that Paul uses several times in the book of Romans is essentially our *physical body* that is leading us into sin as if by instinct. It is as though our body has a mind of its own and forces us to do things against our will when we lash out in anger or reflexively respond in fear.

There is both a biological and a scriptural problem with this position.

Biologically, there is no mechanism that allows our physical body to bypass our brainwaves and engage in complicated tasks related to sin—such as lying, gossiping, slandering, displaying anger—without our mind being involved. In other words, I can find no evidence that our physical body takes us into sin by instinct. However, I have found clear evidence that our choices are influenced by temptation based upon thoughts, feelings, and emotions from Satan's kingdom. Again, when we *feel* angry, afraid, or accused, we often act out sin as we respond to the distressing emotions coming from the enemy's attacks on our minds. Therefore, through the spirit-soul-body connection, it is not the physical body that makes us sin, but the mind receiving lies and temptations from the enemy.

Scripturally, this position that the *flesh* refers to the physical body is based on a misinterpretation of Romans 7:18, "*For I know that in me (that is, in my flesh,) dwelleth no good thing: for to will is present with me; but how to perform that which is good I find not.*"

According to *Strong's Concordance*, this word for "*flesh*" is best defined as "the symbol of what is external."[6] The definition of the flesh as a symbol of something *external to us*—Satan's kingdom—seems to me much more accurate than the opinion that it is our actual physical body. Why? Because, as we stated earlier, our human body does not operate apart from

6. *Strong's* Greek #4561, Knowing Jesus, https://bible.knowing-jesus.com/strongs/G4561.

our soul (mind) when we interact with the world. We make decisions in our soul that produce actions in our body.

Another verse from the apostle Paul that might be misinterpreted by believers concerns the words *"body of sin"* from Romans 6:6, which reads, *"Knowing this, that our old man is crucified with him, that the body of sin might be destroyed, that henceforth we should not serve sin."*

Once again, this *"body of sin"* is not our physical body but Satan's kingdom working on this planet to do evil through humans. How do we know that it does not refer to our physical body? Because God doesn't want our physical body to be destroyed because of sin; He just doesn't want us to serve sin! What must be destroyed is sin, *not* you!

SEPARATION FROM EVIL

At Be in Health, it is our position that although we sin, we are *not* our sin. This key teaching, known as "Separation," helps us understand the spirit-soul-body connection because it addresses evil spirits as being *separate* from your creation—*separate* from who you are. The primary way that Satan's kingdom brings condemnation and confusion into the lives of Christians is by making sin and evil appear to be *one* with us. If we believe that evil thoughts and feelings originate with us, we are stuck with these personality defects and tormenting thoughts. However, if they are from another kingdom, they can be removed by the Holy Spirit, and we can return to peace without them.

Thankfully, the Bible gives us clear evidence that these evil thoughts and feelings do not originate with us but rather originate with the evil spirits that are vexing us in our minds. By recognizing that these thoughts are not our own but are from the enemy, and by repenting of the sin of having embraced these thoughts that are not of God, we can be separated from these evil spirits. Then we can begin the journey of renewing our minds by building new pathways of thought in God's truth, independent of the enemy's evil influence.

Where does our scriptural understanding of the concept of Separation come from? Our primary source is the book of Romans, chapter 7, and Paul's battle with sin. Earlier, in chapter two of this book, we recognized that Paul is describing the believer's battle to overcome sin in our lives. Paul gives us a very honest description of the battle when he confesses that sometimes he does the exact opposite of what he intended to do. During our ministry sessions, there are many attendees who confess they hate being afraid or bitter or angry. They try to avoid manifesting these qualities, and yet, when they are put in certain situations, they do what they do not want to do. This is what Paul describes in Romans 7:15: "*For that which I do I allow not: for what I would, that do I not; but what I hate, that do I.*"

Then, in Romans 17:7, Paul makes another startling statement. It is no longer he that does it *but sin that dwells within him*: "*Now then it is no more I that do it, but sin that dwelleth in me.*"

Therefore, it is our position that sin is not *who we are* but that sin is an evil being. What does that mean? Well, obviously, if we commit sin, it is "our sin" because we allowed evil to manifest through us. If you punch someone, an evil spirit may have manifested through you, but you cannot just blame the devil. You will deal with the consequences of your actions, and sin will be a part of your life. This is part of the bondage and torment humans experience when they embrace the law of sin. Once you repent to Father God and have an evil spirit cast out of you, it is separated from you in order that you might resist its thoughts and feelings in the future and begin to choose to follow God's Word instead.

Let me share an example. We have ministered to many people with anger and rage issues. When they repent of following a spirit of bitterness and anger, we cast it out of them. The result is not necessarily that they will not be tempted to become angry in the future. However, when they are placed in certain situations where they normally would have manifested rage and anger, they do not have those reactions. Instead, they realize that they have a decision to make whether to take an offense or not. This is one of the wonderful miracles of the gospel—to be put into situations where the "old you" would have sinned and to no longer react the same way, to no longer be bound by rage and anger!

Our *separation* from sin is also the point of the message from Genesis 3:11 that we covered in chapter one. What did the Lord ask Adam and Eve after they sinned? "Who told you that you are naked?" By asking this question, I believe that the Lord was challenging Adam and Eve to consider the origin of their thoughts. There was a "who," an evil being, giving Adam and Eve thoughts that were not of God. The feelings and thoughts that caused them to hide from the Lord when their eyes "were opened" were not of God. The feelings they felt once they ate of the forbidden fruit were the result of evil spirits that they had opened themselves up to when they disobeyed God. Simply put, when we disobey God, we open ourselves up to Satan's kingdom.

Part of the problem is that we often define sin as radical actions such as severe drug abuse or physical murder. We may reason that if we haven't committed severely evil acts, we do not have sin in our life. In some cases, we do not acknowledge sin as anything more than an emotional state. For instance, one area of sin many people do not recognize is fear. If the Scriptures clearly state, "Fear not" (see, for example, Isaiah 7:4), isn't this a commandment? Is "Fear not" just a suggestion? No, I consider it sinful to live in fear instead of trusting in Father God. It is not a sin to be startled or taken by surprise, but to live in great fear of people, life's circumstances, or death is sin.

OUR STRUGGLE IS NOT WITH OURSELVES

Please continue tracking with me. The point is, the core of our struggle against sin is not with ourselves but with an evil kingdom determined to destroy our lives. Do not be surprised when you seek to follow Father God and there is another kingdom there to oppose you.

That is why I continue to emphasize this truth: we are tempted through thoughts, feelings, and emotions from Satan's kingdom because he is determined to make us believe that we are evil, to convince us that sin is a part of us. A spirit of bitterness wants you to believe you are *a bitter person* and that it is a part of your original thought process. A spirit of fear will make you feel afraid and lead you to the conclusion that you are just *a fearful person.* These evil spirits want you to believe that they are *you!* Many humans associate themselves with these negative attributes, and they will describe themselves as being a fearful person or an angry person. The problem is that you have made Satan's nature part of your personality. We need these sins to be purified out of our lives so that we may be overcomers, so that we may be free.

I find then a law, that, when I would do good, evil is present with me. For I delight in the law of God after the inward man: but I see another law in my members, warring against the law of my mind, and bringing me into captivity to the law of sin which is in my members. O wretched man that I am! who shall deliver me from the body of this death? I thank God through Jesus Christ our Lord. So then with the mind I myself serve the law of God; but with the flesh the law of sin.

(Romans 7:21–25)

TEMPTATION IS NOT SIN

We are caught between two kingdoms and must decide which one we will follow. Regardless of the thoughts we have or even our feelings of fear, anger, or otherwise, we need to make the decision to trust the Word of God despite these temptations.

I want you to understand that temptation is *not* sin. I clearly defined the pathways of beta, alpha, and theta brainwaves to help you understand how Satan's kingdom speaks to you. It may often feel like you have sinned or done something wrong because you had an evil thought, but just because that thought passed through your mind, it does not mean you sinned. It could just be temptation from evil spirits. If you have been listening to these thoughts and following them for years, do not feel condemned; you do not need to stay there. Repent to Father God for following these thoughts and feelings. Embrace the freedom of His forgiveness and His love for you.

Some individuals wish for temptation to disappear so that they can be at peace to follow the Bible. The truth of the matter is you must make a decision to follow Father God despite feeling angry or fearful. You need to choose to follow either Satan's kingdom or the kingdom of God. The choice is up to you.

THE 8 RS TO FREEDOM

At Be in Health, we teach what we call the 8 Rs to Freedom.[7] As we move into specific roots of disease, it is essential that you be aware of these concepts, especially the first 4 Rs. As we shine a light on spiritual problems, you will need to recognize the problem, repent to Father God, and renounce the evil influence on your life. The final 4 Rs are also essential and represent your future freedom. When you are bound to evil spirits they must be removed, then you must learn to resist them. The final two represent extending God's kingdom in your life and others' lives. Rejoice in your freedom and restore others as you have been restored. It is vital for you to remember and apply them. Post them where you can see them daily, such as on your refrigerator or on your bathroom mirror. Most important, post them on your heart. They are the pathway to your freedom!

1. **Recognize.** *You must recognize what it is.* Recognize the root problem(s) in your life: bitterness, hatred, fear, anxiety, anger, hostility, self-hatred, etc. Pray for discernment from the Holy Spirit. Discern good from evil in your life.

2. **Responsibility.** *You must take responsibility for what you recognize.* Not everybody wants to take responsibility after they recognize the problem. You need to take responsibility. God will walk alongside you, but He won't do it for you!

3. **Repent.** *Repent to God of participating in what you recognize.* The Bible tells us, *"Repent ye therefore, and be converted, that your sins may be blotted out, when the times of refreshing shall come from the presence of the Lord"* (Acts 3:19). Some people get mad at me when I tell them they need to repent to be free from disease. If you go to a doctor to find out why you are sick and how to get better, would you be offended if he told you the truth? No? Then please do not be offended if I tell you the truth. I love you; I care what happens to you, and I'm teaching you how to defeat evil spirits and disease.

4. **Renounce.** *You must make what you recognize your enemy and renounce it.* To repent literally means "to turn away from." Consider your past root of sin as your enemy—and renounce it! Some

7. Dr. Henry W. Wright, *A More Excellent Way* (New Kensington, PA: Whitaker House, 2009), 161–169.

people have remorse, but they do not change on the inside. They don't turn away from their sin. But I want you to get away from evil—as fast as you can. Love yourself—but hate the evil!

5. **Remove it. *Get rid of it once and for all!*** Say to the law of sin within you, "Not only do I renounce you, but you and I cannot exist at the same place and the same time together. *"Cast away from you all your transgressions, whereby ye have transgressed; and make you a new heart and a new spirit"* (Ezekiel 18:31). Get that law of sin out of your face, and let God give you a new heart and spirit.

6. **Resist. *When it tries to come back, resist it!*** James 4:7 tells us that we are to submit ourselves to God and resist the devil: *"Submit yourselves therefore to God. Resist the devil, and he will flee from you."* Which one comes first? Submitting to God. Only then will you have the power to resist the enemy, not before. Whatever you have dealt with will try to come back. That is why we need God and each other to resist it.

7. **Rejoice. *Give God thanks for setting you free.*** Give God glory for your freedom! Praise Him that you have experienced grace and mercy from a living God who loves you. He is worthy of your praise!

8. **Restore. *Help someone else get free.*** After you have received the blessings of God, it's time for you to begin helping to restore others. Part of restoring is bringing the gospel to those you love, instructing those who are separated from the refreshing of the Lord, and discipling them in freedom from disease. *"There should be no schism in the body; but that the members should have the same care for one another. And whether one member suffer, all the members suffer with it; or one member be honoured, all the members rejoice with it"* (1 Corinthians 12:25–26).

TAKING THOUGHTS CAPTIVE

It is not sin to feel temptation in the form of thoughts and feelings, but it is important to consider what we will do with these thoughts and feelings after we are set free. Once you have repented of the sin of believing the enemy's lies and have those spirits cast out of you, what should you do with the thoughts that he still brings to your mind to compete with God's Word? Second Corinthians 10:4–5 reveals spiritual weapons that are a key to overcoming thoughts from the enemy.

(For the weapons of our warfare are not carnal, but mighty through God to the pulling down of strong holds;) casting down imaginations, and every high thing that exalteth itself against the knowledge of God, and bringing into captivity every thought to the obedience of Christ.
(2 Corinthians 10:4–5)

We are to "cast down imaginations and every high thing that exalts itself against the knowledge of God." What does that mean? Satan's tempting thoughts are "imaginations" and "high things" that exalt themselves against God's knowledge found in the Bible. How do we cast them down? This is how you can handle it: in one hand, hold up what Satan says through temptation, and in the other hand, lift up what God says in His Word to contradict Satan. Then, take Satan's lie and cast it down in the name of Jesus.

What does "bringing into captivity to the obedience of Christ" mean? It means even if you feel fearful, angry, or otherwise, do not follow those thoughts but choose to follow the Word of God despite what you feel. The world that is following Satan's kingdom is being taught to go with their feelings. We are taught to follow the Word of God *despite* our feelings. This process has nothing to do with our emotions, but it has everything to do with our freedom, which comes from embracing the truth of God's Word.

HEALED IN SPIRIT, SOUL, AND BODY

JANICE

As a young mother at just twenty-six years old, I began a painful journey of disease. First came the diagnosis of sarcoidosis, an interconnective tissue disease that attacks your organs. It attacked my lungs, and the doctors had to biopsy my liver and spine, as well. I lost a lot of weight, was very weak and tired, and had breathing issues. In the years following, I was hit with one autoimmune diagnosis after the other—interstitial cystitis, lichen sclerosis, hypoglycemia—and they were all considered incurable.

I carried these illnesses, along with others, throughout my young adult years, managing them as best I could with medical help, until I was in my early fifties and my daughter gave me Dr. Henry Wright's book *A More Excellent Way*. I started reading it and was amazed that it was filled with answers of hope for me. The thing that stood out to me the most, though, was something I had a hard time wrapping my head around. I had been a Christian for years, but I had never heard about the devastating results that self-hatred and self-loathing can do to our bodies. My husband and I, along with our daughter, made an appointment to see Dr. Wright when he was speaking at a conference in Sarasota, Florida. That was my first giant step toward wholeness—spirit, soul, and body.

The following year, my husband and I attended a For My Life retreat and learned about the spiritual roots of autoimmune disease and so many other things that affect us when we accept the lies of the enemy instead of embracing the truth of God's Word. I hadn't realized how important this was to our health and wholeness. I began to apply so many things to my life that I had never been taught in church—about the Father's love for me, and how important it is for me to love myself.

In addition to the autoimmune diseases, I also suffered with fibromyalgia, a stress disorder that brings pain in your muscles and ligaments, along with fatigue and insomnia. I learned that the spiritual root of fibromyalgia was from carrying so much fear and anxiety because of a father who wasn't really present for me, and then from my husband who was very driven. The spirits of fear, drivenness to perform to earn love, and guilt—I took it all on as I believed the enemy's lies. At For My Life, I learned how important it was to be easy on myself and not be driven to perform for those around me.

I believe that the prayers of deliverance over my life were also vital. I was delivered of the spirits of self-hatred, self-resentment, self-bitterness, fear, and rejection. I know that was a key to my healing and recovery. I've also been delivered from the spirit of death and the spirit of infirmity. The enemy was after me. He stole from me for over twenty-five years of my life, but God is the great restorer!

Praise God, after the For My Life retreat, I was set free of the fibromyalgia almost immediately. Being healed from the autoimmune diseases didn't happen as quickly. It took three or four more years before my healing was complete with all my symptoms gone. Since I had dwelt on the enemy's lies of self-hate for over twenty-five years, I needed to dwell continuously on God's Word and allow it to transform how I felt about myself, to transform how I understood God's love for me.

I read Psalm 139 regularly, that I was fearfully and wonderfully made. I studied Psalm 103:3, that God forgives all of my sins and heals all of my diseases. Well, if I believe that God forgives all my sins, why don't I believe He can heal all my diseases? I began to believe that He could. I also meditated on Jesus's command that I must not only love God with all of me, but that I must love myself. (See Mark 12:30–31.) I finally understood that

God's perfect will is not just to heal me but to keep me walking in health. And during that time, every one of those autoimmune symptoms disappeared. I was healed and free!

I've been in the church since I was in my twenties. I was prayed for and anointed with oil many times, but I was not healed until I started believing and applying the Word of God. Jesus is my Healer. I had to believe that. When we went to For My Life, I saw it modeled before me, and I realized it was truth. It increased my faith that there's more to God and His plans than I knew. I wanted to know the more.

Today, over fifteen years since the last symptom disappeared, I am still free of all of it. I'm seventy-one, and I have more energy than I did when I was a young mother. I had a lot of brain fog back then, which is completely gone. My ability to function in every way is mine. I've got my life back. Free from all of it. My husband and I have been pastoring a church for the last fourteen years, where we share the power of the Word of God, including how He makes us whole—spirit, soul, and body!

FIVE

PATHWAYS OF DISEASE

I had some personal experience with the spirit-soul-body connection very early in my ministry. I was young, pastoring my first church in Florida. We met in a storefront, and that included Monday night prayer meetings.

One Monday, the prayer meeting had just begun when a young woman from the church pulled up in front of the building and ran inside, saying, "We're on the way to the emergency room! I know you're having a prayer meeting, and I want to give God a chance first." She continued, "My husband is experiencing some kind of involuntary muscle spasm! He is shaking all over and falling to the floor! We don't know what to do!"

I ran out to the sidewalk and yanked open the passenger door of the car. Her husband was half in the seat and half on the floor, shaking violently. It was so startling that the first thing that came out of my mouth was, "Whoa!"

In those early days of ministry, I was at the start of my journey to understand disease. "What are you going to do with that?" I thought to myself. "Call 9-1-1" was the logical answer. But I stopped to pray first instead. "Father," I said, "I haven't the foggiest idea what's going on, but You do."

I had been a pre-med student in college, so I had some knowledge of the human body. One word jumped into my mind as soon as I prayed: *hypothalamus*. I found myself praying, "I take authority over the spirit of fear that's giving signals to the hypothalamus to produce this involuntary muscle spasm. I command the spirit of fear to be gone and the hypothalamus not to take any more information from that spirit of fear. Central nervous system, be at peace; muscle spasms, stop now, in Jesus's name." And just like that, it stopped. Her husband sat up on the passenger seat, and she drove him home. We went back into the prayer meeting in awe of what God had just done.

LAUNCHING A JOURNEY

When I got home later that night, I had some serious questions for the Lord. "God, what happened tonight? Why did I say 'hypothalamus'? What's the hypothalamus?" I had studied that part of the brain somewhat in those pre-med years, but so what? I got out a textbook from college on pathophysiology and began to read what the hypothalamus does.

I was shocked to realize that I had spoken accurately to the spirit that had taken over this man's mind with feelings and thoughts that had caused him to become fearful. This had triggered the hypothalamus gland to begin producing neurological misfirings, causing the involuntary muscle spasms that had him on the floor of his car. I had prayed accurately, and I didn't have the foggiest idea why. But I learned a never-forgotten lesson that night: God has given us a connection between the spirit, the soul, and the body.

That incident launched my journey to study the connection between thought and physiology. The result of my studies are tens of thousands of people worldwide who now have the knowledge for their freedom from disease, and thousands who are being healed from the diseases they have been battling.

It is my desire to pass along this knowledge to you, as well. Some of the details are a little technical, but please keep tracking with me. It is for your life and your health!

YOU ARE A MIRACLE!

God has created the human body with a plan for your health. You need to understand how your body is constructed—and how God's plan can be thwarted by the decisions you make in your thought life. We'll start at your beginning.

Shortly after conception, the fertilized egg begins the process of cell mitosis, which is simply the original cells multiplying into additional formative cells. Three of the earliest cells in your body development form the ectoderm, the mesoderm, and the endoderm. What are they? Amazing foundational blocks for the development of the entire human body. Again, please follow along with me because these details are important for overcoming disease.

Take a close look at chart 2 on the following page. There you are. Developed from the ectoderm, you have a brain, a nervous system, a cardiovascular system, a heart rhythm, skin, hair, eyes, ears, and a nose. From the mesoderm, you have your heart circulation, muscles, skeletal form, kidneys, bone marrow, blood vessels, lymph glands, and more. Finally, from the endoderm, you have your liver, lungs, intestines, urinary tract, and endocrine system, which includes important glands such as the pituitary and hypothalamus glands.

This is you. This is what you are on the inside past the gorgeous hunk of dust looking at us! You are a creative miracle! And all of these systems are highly responsive and regulated by a flow that originates in your brain.

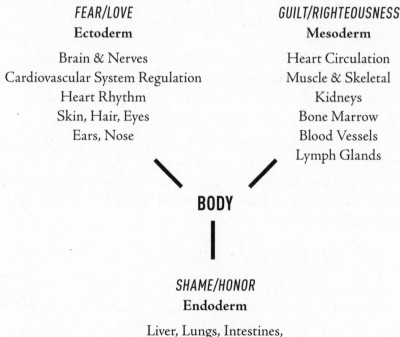

FEAR/LOVE
Ectoderm

Brain & Nerves
Cardiovascular System Regulation
Heart Rhythm
Skin, Hair, Eyes
Ears, Nose

GUILT/RIGHTEOUSNESS
Mesoderm

Heart Circulation
Muscle & Skeletal
Kidneys
Bone Marrow
Blood Vessels
Lymph Glands

BODY

SHAME/HONOR
Endoderm

Liver, Lungs, Intestines,
Urinary, Endocrine

Chart 2

YOUR BRAIN AND YOUR NERVOUS SYSTEM

You have two parts to your nervous system. The first is the voluntary nervous system, giving you control over your bodily movements. You can tell your arm to raise and your hand to scratch your head when you want to. Then, you have the involuntary or sympathetic nervous system, which God created so that your body functions without having to think about it. This is how your heart pumps, you breathe, and your digestive organs work.

Now, if you have a long-term memory full of thoughts that oppose God's Word, you can interfere with both the voluntary and involuntary nervous systems and cause them to function improperly; that is what I call the *dis-ease* of function. If you have embraced the enemy's thoughts for years, your body systems will malfunction because they are without peace or *without ease*. Dis-ease is exactly what it sounds like: the lack of ease or health within your spirit and your body's systems.

Stay with me here as we go a little further. In chart 3, we are looking at the brain. Your limbic system is the part of the brain that deals with your emotions and your memory. There are four main parts in the limbic system, but to understand the roots of disease, I want to focus on two in particular: the amygdalae glands and the hypothalamus gland.

The amygdalae glands located in your brain are responsible for what we call the "fight-or-flight" reaction to emergency situations, stress, and fear. The amygdalae also play a vital role in storing our long-term memories. The amygdalae are involved in our deeply felt emotions, whether negative (like panic and anger) or positive (like love and laughter).

Tracking Fear in the Brain

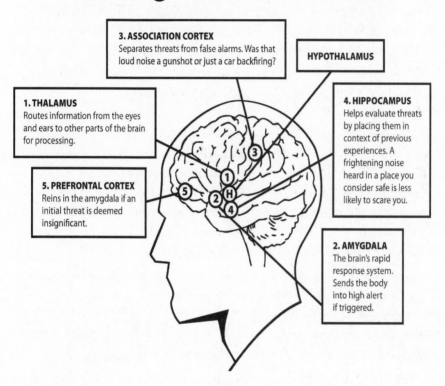

3. ASSOCIATION CORTEX
Separates threats from false alarms. Was that loud noise a gunshot or just a car backfiring?

HYPOTHALAMUS

1. THALAMUS
Routes information from the eyes and ears to other parts of the brain for processing.

4. HIPPOCAMPUS
Helps evaluate threats by placing them in context of previous experiences. A frightening noise heard in a place you consider safe is less likely to scare you.

5. PREFRONTAL CORTEX
Reins in the amygdala if an initial threat is deemed insignificant.

2. AMYGDALA
The brain's rapid response system. Sends the body into high alert if triggered.

Chart 3

THE HYPOTHALAMUS: A SMALL GLAND WITH A BIG JOB

Now, let's look at the importance of the pea-sized gland called the hypothalamus. This gland is very significant to our understanding of the spiritual roots of disease. We are now going to expose the specific biological pathway that Satan uses to bring disease.

Let's look at chart 4 to see what the hypothalamus gland controls. Your endocrine system is a chemical messenger system that involves several important glands in your body, including the pituitary gland, the adrenal glands, and the hypothalamus gland. These glands secrete hormones that keep your body balanced and working smoothly. Of these glands, the hypothalamus is considered the control center of the entire endocrine system. It is a small but vital gland in the center of your brain.

The main role of the hypothalamus is to keep your body in homeostasis, which means in a healthy body balance. It regulates the other glands, telling them when they should secrete the hormones that are necessary for your body to remain in homeostasis. Your body works continually to maintain this balance because, without it, you will develop a disorder or disease.

Endocrine System

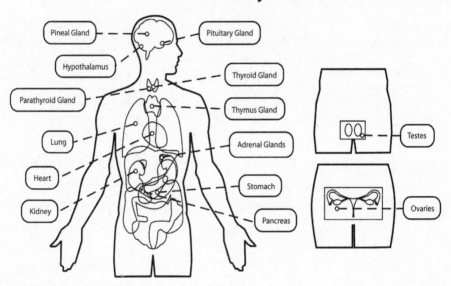

Chart 4

THE MASTER CONTROL

As the master control, the hypothalamus regulates many bodily activities: body temperature, thirst, appetite and weight control, emotions, sleep cycles, sex drive, childbirth, blood pressure and heart rate, production of digestive juices, and balancing of body fluids. It activates your thyroid, which, in turn, affects your metabolism, energy levels, and developmental growth. It stirs the pituitary gland to release growth hormones.

The hypothalamus is working continually, controlling the release of hormones from the other endocrine glands to maintain homeostasis in all of these systems. For example, if it receives a message that you are too hot, it will trigger the appropriate gland to produce sweat. If it receives the message that you are too cold, it will create heat through shivering. As a result, unless you are sick, your body maintains a stable body temperature.

Since the hypothalamus regulates your heart rate, the contraction of your heart muscles, and the movement of food through the digestive system, serious problems occur when it is not functioning normally. An interference in the function of your cardiovascular system can cause high blood pressure and heart attacks. In the gastrointestinal system, disorders can result in such things as ulcerative colitis, irritable bowel syndrome, diarrhea, vomiting, and nausea.

WHAT YOU MEDITATE ON REGULATES THE HYPOTHALAMUS

The hypothalamus plays a central role in the spirit-soul-body connection that we have been discussing. The cerebral cortex covers the largest part of the brain. It is how we process information, thinking, language comprehension, problem solving, and—most important for this study— long-term memory. When you are meditating on—or continually replaying—thoughts of fear, anxiety, bitterness, anger, or self-hatred, the amygdalae receive and interpret those strong negative emotions and thoughts as a threat. The rest of the limbic system kicks into survival mode, and the hypothalamus gland responds.

As the hypothalamus receives these messages, it may become overwhelmed. The result may be hypoactivity or hyperactivity in the endocrine system, neurological misfiring, and neurotransmitter imbalance. Your thoughts, and the evil spirit behind them, have disrupted the hypothalamus's proper function. Over time, living this way can lead to serious destruction of your body and organs.

In chart 5, you can see the list of diseases that result from a lack of homeostasis. It will affect the gastrointestinal system and create sexual disorders (impotence and frigidity), skin diseases (eczema, neurodermatitis, acne), diabetes, fatigue and lethargy, overeating, depression, and insomnia. In addition, it can lead to coronary artery disease, hypertension, stroke, disturbances of heart rhythm, tension headaches, muscle contractions, backaches, rheumatoid arthritis, related inflammatory diseases, asthma, hay fever, immunosuppression, and autoimmune disease—all stemming from a dysfunction of the hypothalamus gland that creates a lack of homeostasis.

EXAMPLES OF STRESS-RELATED DISEASES AND CONDITIONS

TARGET ORGAN OR SYSTEM	DISEASE OR CONDITION
Cardiovascular System	• Coronary artery disease • Hypertension • Stroke • Disturbances of heart rhythm
Muscles	• Tension headaches • Muscle contraction backache
Connective Tissues	• Rheumatoid arthritis (autoimmune disease) • Related inflammatory diseases of connective tissue
Pulmonary System	• Asthma (hypersensitivity reaction) • Hay fever (hypersensitivity reaction)
Immune System	• Immunosuppressant or deficiency • Autoimmune diseases
Gastrointestinal System	• Ulcer • Irritable bowel syndrome • Diarrhea • Nausea and vomiting • Ulcerative colitis
Genitourinary System	• Diuresis • Impotence • Frigidity
Skin	• Eczema • Neurodermatitis • Acne
Endocrine System	• Diabetes mellitus • Amenorrhea
Central Nervous System	• Fatigue and lethargy • Type A behavior • Overeating • Depression • Insomnia

Chart 5

Our research at Be in Health comes from studying what the medical and scientific community understands about our body. They see how the hypothalamus responds to our emotions. As I assured you earlier, I am not an enemy of science. Look at the information it has provided for our understanding of the physical function of our bodies.

Science confirms that there is a direct correspondence between anxiety and heart palpitations.[8] There's a direct correspondence between hostility and coronary artery thrombosis.[9] There's a direct connection between shame and irritable bowel syndrome.[10]

THE HYPOTHALAMUS IS THE PATHWAY THE ENEMY USES

Now, how is our spirit-man involved in this connection between the mind, the hypothalamus gland, and disease? Remember, the soul (the mind and emotions) is the bridge between the spirit world and the physical world. Father God, through His Word, provides peace for our spirit first. When we obey His Word, then our soul and body can come into homeostasis. On the other hand, the devil uses temptation in our thought life to get us to disobey God's Word, leading to imbalance, or dis-ease, in our bodies.

If the hypothalamus can be triggered into dysfunction through temptations—and if a lack of homeostasis can cause disease—then the enemy has a clear pathway to bring disease into our lives, doesn't he? Here is the pathway:

1. The enemy tempts us with thoughts that oppose the Word of God—thoughts of unrighteousness, such as unforgiveness, bitterness, self-hatred, greed, envy, jealousy, anger, hostility, fear, stress, and anxiety. These are part of the law of sin.

2. If we embrace those unrighteous thoughts and meditate or dwell on them instead of on the Word of God, they become a part of our long-term memory and a part of our biology.

---

8. P. Tyler and D. Baldwin, "Generalised Anxiety Disorder," *Lancet* 368 (2006): 2156–2166.
9. Daichi Shimbo et al., "Hostility and Platelet Reactivity in Individuals Without a History of Cardiovascular Disease Events," *Psychosomatic Medicine* 71 (2009): 741–747.
10. D. A. Drossman et al., "A Focus Group Assessment of Patient Perspectives on Irritable Bowel Syndrome and Illness Severity," *Digestive Diseases and Sciences* 54 (2009): 1532–1541.

3. These elevated negative emotions, and the spirits behind them, are communicated from the amygdalae and the cerebral cortex to the hypothalamus gland, which then triggers the wrong signals to other vital glands in our body. If we live this way day to day, it can damage our bodies over time. As a result of living in sin and with a lack of homeostasis, we may develop serious diseases, including heart disease, cancer, rheumatoid arthritis, diabetes, and so many more.

What a devious plan of the enemy! Think about it. The hypothalamus is the only gland that Satan and his kingdom need to move you in the direction of disease! Instead of our body functioning as God intended, we have dis-ease of function. If that dis-ease continues, it can develop into a full-blown disorder or disease.

Satan understands how the human body functions. The enemy just needs that one gland to set this whole mess in motion. He understands what he needs to do to send it into imbalance and to wreak havoc with our health. He is good at it—but God is so much bigger. That is why I am laying out the knowledge for you to know how to fight Satan's plan of disease for your life. Do not dwell on the enemy's evil temptations. Instead, meditate on the truth in God's Word.

I want you to have victory over the enemy's plan! I am passionate about this because your life and health are at stake. There is a zeal burning in me to get this message out to as many people as possible. Church, it's time to wake up! Salvation is here. I pray for the Holy Spirit to awaken your spirit and soul to this spiritual and physical threat. I pray that all believers may embrace this truth for themselves and their loved ones.

HEALED OF LUPUS

LAUREN

I have had some incredible healing. Back in 2013, I was going through terrible symptoms because of lupus. I was in and out of the hospital several times, my kidneys weren't working properly, and I had terrible joint swelling over my entire body. I couldn't even make a fist or bend my arms fully because my joints were constantly swollen. I had the lupus butterfly rash on my face and had visible bumps around my joints because of the inflammation.

When I received the lupus diagnosis, I didn't want to believe it. I was given medication, but it didn't help. The doctors told me that the torch had been lit; there was no cure, and I would have lupus for the rest of my life. I walked out of the office and into the hallway, and before I even left the building, I called my sister, Anne, and told her, "I refuse to accept this diagnosis."

Soon after, I went to a For My Life retreat, and over time, by applying the biblical principles I learned there, I gradually got better. I can now say that I am completely healed of lupus!

What is even more amazing is that I recently had my first child, a baby boy. When I still had the lupus, my doctors told me that I was at a high risk for pregnancy complications. Even though my lupus was healed, during my pregnancy I had to have weekly ultrasounds for twelve weeks in a row. Each time, I got good news from the doctors that my baby was fine.

I feel so incredibly blessed that I was healed of lupus and that I was able to have a healthy child. Now, I am even back to doing my gymnastics and waterskiing. My health has been fully restored. Doctors rarely see healings happen like this, so my rheumatologist asked me to still come in periodically for blood tests. It's been two years now, and every time they test me, I have normal results. Thank You, God.

My healing didn't happen instantly but rather in a journey over time. God does heal instantly, but keep an open mind that it can also be a successful journey.

SIX

THE SPIRITUAL ROOTS OF ALLERGIES

According to the U.S. Centers for Disease Control and Prevention, allergies are the sixth leading cause of chronic illness in the U.S.[11]

If you look up a definition of allergies on the Internet, you will find an answer like this: "An allergy is an abnormal reaction by your immune system to a substance that is usually not harmful." What kinds of substances? Pollen, animal fur, flowers, perfumes, peanuts, eggs, milk products, shellfish, fibers, and more. Having allergies means you are allergic to God's creation, things He meant for you to enjoy. That is not God's plan.

Doctors and researchers aren't sure why some people get allergies, and they do not believe allergies can be cured—only managed by medication and lifestyle changes. Here we go again! The medical community does not understand the root cause of a disease or disorder, so they just manage the symptoms with antihistamines and other medicines.

By God's grace, we have had great results over the last thirty years with people being completely healed of their allergies. I believe that God has shown us the root cause that truly lies behind allergies. It is my intention to unfold this revelation by looking at what medicine says, as well as what we have discovered through For My Life that has brought restoration and healing to many, many lives.

---

11. "Allergy Facts," American College of Allergy, Asthma and Immunology, https://acaai.org/news/facts-statistics/allergies.

THE SPIRIT OF FEAR AND STRESS

Have you ever been fearful? Have you ever seen a fearful person? Apart from horror movies, you might answer, "No." More relatable questions would be: Have you ever been stressed out? Have you ever seen a stressed-out person before? What does it look and feel like? A person may feel tension in their neck; it may manifest in a headache, irritability, or scrambled, scattered thinking.

Now, have you ever considered what causes stress? Is it possible that stress is the result of being afraid? Young children often respond to fear in very obvious ways. If they see a spider, for instance, they might scream and run away; certainly, adults may do the same! On the other hand, as an adult you probably have more complicated fears. Many of us spend all our time being fearful about our job, our finances, our relationships, and even our health.

We may say we are not afraid, we are just "stressed out" about these issues. I would like to show you that, according to Scripture, stress and fear are synonymous! When you are stressed out, would you say you are at peace? No. You are probably tormented by your thoughts, as well. They replay in your mind; you can't escape them. People who are stressed out often have trouble sleeping at night because the stressful thoughts do not end just because it is time to go to bed. According to 1 John 4:18, these indicators point to the fact that many people who feel stressed are actually fearful.

There is no fear in love; but perfect love casteth out fear: because fear hath torment. He that feareth is not made perfect in love.

(1 John 4:18)

The purpose of pointing all this out is to identify the spiritual defect behind "stress." It is a spirit of fear. Remember, we are not talking about an emotion of fear but an evil *spirit of fear* that manifests as stress in our human minds and bodies. *"For God hath not given us the spirit of fear; but of power, and of love, and of a sound mind"* (2 Timothy 1:7).

Many modern Bible translations have changed the wording of 2 Timothy 1:7. They have replaced the phrase *"spirit of fear"* with the word "timidity," omitting the word *spirit* altogether. This change removes the spiritual discernment of recognizing there is an evil spirit and replaces it with an emotional descriptor of timidity. By altering this Scripture, we may no longer recognize that it is the evil spirit of fear that tempts and controls us.

In the Old Testament, the book of Job also identifies fear as a spirit:

Fear came upon me, and trembling, which made all my bones to shake. Then a spirit passed before my face; the hair of my flesh stood up: it stood still, but I could not discern the form thereof: an image was before mine eyes, there was silence, and I heard a voice, saying....

(Job 4:14–16)

Fear is not just a psychological manifestation; it is an evil spirit that is plotting against us. The spirit of fear comes from Satan's hidden kingdom. God is the One who calls it the spirit of fear. We would be wise not to disagree with Him.

Hebrews, chapter 11, opens with a strong statement about faith: *"Now faith is the substance of things hoped for, the evidence of things not seen"* (Hebrews 11:1). On the opposite side of faith, fear is the substance of things we *do not hope for!* Fear is a powerful aspect of Satan's belief system. While faith is greater than fear, they are equal in these two ways: they both project into the future, and they both demand to be fulfilled. Jesus said, *"According to your faith be it unto you"* (Matthew 9:29). The enemy wants to replace that with, "According to your fear be it unto you!"

We know that science recognizes some of the results of fear. Most medical professionals agree that having a fearful outlook on life will cause your health to be affected negatively. Allergies are a product or a result of who you are deep within and how you relate to God, yourself, and others, rather than primarily how your body responds to the natural environment around you. Many people don't want to hear this, but I believe all allergies are caused by the spirit of fear.

Psalm 34:4 says, "*I sought the* LORD, *and he heard me, and delivered me from all my fears.*" There is hope. If we seek the Lord and call upon His name, we will be delivered. That's a promise we need to embrace.

THE RESULTS OF FEAR ON YOUR IMMUNE SYSTEM

What happens if we embrace fear instead of faith and allow the spirit of fear to control our lives? To answer this question, I am going to show you, from both a spiritual and medical standpoint, what causes allergies.

First, let's talk about cortisol. Cortisol is a naturally occurring steroid released by the adrenal glands. It has its function, especially to help us in fight-or-flight situations that could be dangerous. But if cortisol is released unchecked, it becomes a "cortisol drip." Cortisol drip is the term I use to help you understand how this release of cortisol acts—like a leaky faucet. It is continually being released. If you continue to manifest anxiety and stress in your life, then the drip, drip of cortisol will begin to weaken your immune system.

Now, I am not referring to a phobic fear such as fear of flying or fear of spiders. This fear predominantly results from relationship breakdowns. The primary spiritual cause of allergies is a spirit of fear related to not feeling safe in love and relationships. The result is additional fear and anxiety in all relationships. It will cause you to avoid or push others away for fear that they will injure or harm you. This spirit of fear will also lead you into isolation. Cortisol does not destroy the immune system because of nutrition. *Cortisol destroys the immune system because of a spirit of fear.*

A COMPROMISED IMMUNE SYSTEM

You might be shocked to learn you are not really allergic to anything. You are experiencing the biological phenomenon of fear and the consequences of cortisol release. You are experiencing a biological manifestation that results in a compromised immune system.

The immune system is the part of your body that God created to identify organisms that are dangerous to you and to destroy them. God has created several different types of white corpuscles to be fully formed, ready for action and ready for war. For the purposes of this chapter, I want to focus on the white corpuscles called the T cells and the B cells. If you have a healthy immune system, nothing foreign can stand in their path. However, there are various things that can interfere with your immune system, keeping it from serving you. Excessive cortisol is one of them.

When Cortisol is Oversecreted

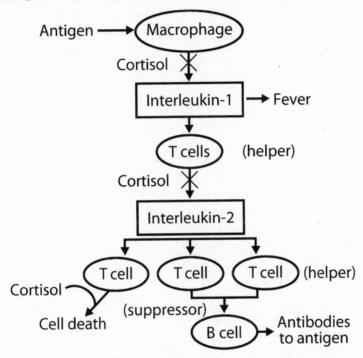

Chart 6

Take a look at chart 6. If cortisol is drip, drip, dripping, the result is the death of T cells. Some T cells serve as killer cells, attacking and destroying viruses and other invaders. Other T cells are assigned to suppress B cell activity once the foreign invader has been neutralized. B cells produce antibodies that also act like killer cells and destroy the invaders.

WHEN THE SYSTEM BREAKS DOWN

Here's what happens when things go wrong. As the immune system is compromised by the cortisol drip, the T cells that help to guide the work of the immune system are destroyed by the cortisol. At the same time, the B cell activity increases and becomes excessive. Every cell in your body, healthy cells and invader cells—including viruses, bacteria, and cancer—has an identifying marker called an antigen flag. When things function the way God created them to, the antibodies recognize the antigen flags and attack and destroy the unhealthy invaders.

Unfortunately, when your immune system is malfunctioning, this system has a breakdown. The B cells mistakenly create antibodies that attack the antigen markers of natural substances that are not invaders. Instead of attacking viruses and bacteria, they will attack grass, pollen, dust, animal fur, perfumes, and certain foods. Your body reacts with an overproduction of histamine, which produces various "allergic" reactions, such as itchy eyes, runny nose, sinus headaches, and rashes. You can take an antihistamine to get some relief from the symptoms, but it doesn't make the problem go away.

To the degree that your T cell activity decreases, B cell activity increases. That is why the more your immune system is compromised, the more complicated your allergies become, from simple to medium to complex. If your immune system is normal, B cell activity is regulated, and allergies cease to exist. You can be around anything and be able to eat anything you want and never react. To recap, an allergy is the result of fear, anxiety, and stress, which causes excessive B cell activity from T cell death coming out of long-term cortisol drip.

WHAT IS THE SECRET TO DEFEATING ALLERGIES?

When a person comes to us with allergies, we do not need to do any bloodwork. We know that person has a compromised immune system. The number of allergies you have tells me how badly your immune system is compromised. I have seen as many as one hundred allergies leave a person's body in twenty-four hours, never to return. Thousands of people around the world no longer have allergies, not because of my anointing for healing, but because of the truth of this information. People who were locked away in foil-lined rooms, allergic to foods, smells, perfumes, and many other things, are living normal lives today.

What is the secret to defeating allergies? Recognize the fear that is causing the release of cortisol. Repent of the spirit of fear manifesting as stress and anxiety in your soul/mind and body, and God will give you a blood transfusion at the marrow level. God loves you. Receive His love and allow Him to deliver you from your fears. Begin to accept yourself and love yourself again. Renew your mind in God's Word as you learn to trust in and rely on Him. Mend the broken relationships in your life that have caused the fear. Forgive the person or persons who may have led to your distrust and fear of relationships. When your immune system is healed, your allergies will be a thing of the past.

HOW TO KEEP YOUR IMMUNE SYSTEM HEALTHY

Doctors know about cortisol and what it does to the body when it goes drip, drip, drip. So, why can't they help you with this drip? The medical community uses vitamins, herbs, and health food to try to build up your immune system. But, remember, the source isn't nutritional problems. The source is a spirit of fear. Then, doctors give you more fear about eating the wrong foods. My question to them is, "Why are you still doing something that isn't working?" It is fear that creates the overabundance of cortisol that destroys the immune system. We are creating prisons for people, not places of freedom.

How do you keep your immune system healthy? Allow Father God to develop His nature in you. God's nature includes the nine fruit of the Spirit, which are given to us in the fifth chapter of Galatians: *"The fruit of the Spirit is love, joy, peace, longsuffering, gentleness, goodness, faith, meekness, temperance: against such there is no law"* (Galatians 5:22–23).

The Holy Spirit is the third member of the Godhead and represents Father God's nature, among other things. Therefore, to have an immune system that is like the one God intends you to have, your nature should express love, joy, peace, longsuffering, gentleness, goodness, faithfulness, kindness, and temperance! The Bible says that there is no law that can defeat this fruit! This nature of God in you is what produces a healthy immune system.

I want you to win this battle! For the sake of your health, get rid of as much fear as you can because God is not giving it to you; the enemy is. Let the Holy Spirit form His incredible nature in you. The enemy might still tempt you, but he cannot touch you. Take ownership of your life!

ADDRESSING SIMPLE ALLERGIES AND CHILDREN

Some time ago, I was holding a conference in New England, and two very concerned parents brought their baby boy to me with a severe case of eczema that covered half of his face. The little guy was under a year old, and doctors had prescribed as many antihistamines and topical creams as they could, but nothing was helping. In most cases with skin allergies of this type, medical professionals will give you a topical application and an antihistamine. But what is the root cause of the problem? The parents asked me, "What can we do?"

That day, I looked those parents straight in the eyes and asked, "Is it possible that one of you is struggling to love and accept your child just the way he is?" I opened up a real can of worms there. In such circumstances, I don't intend to be mean. I don't intend to be accusatory. But lives are at stake.

The mother burst into tears on the spot and confessed that she was the one who was struggling in this way. This was a Christian mom. While she was pregnant, she had her heart set on having a girl. When her son was born, she wasn't excited about bonding with him or nurturing him. She was reluctant to breastfeed him and rarely snuggled him. The baby didn't understand any of it; he couldn't even understand words yet. All the child responded to was physical touch or the lack of it.

The mother of this child was convicted. She didn't realize what she had been doing, that her actions had been a way of not accepting her baby. She cried out to God and repented for rejecting the child. Then, she snuggled that baby boy, and, with tears streaming down, repented to him, asking him to forgive her. Even though he couldn't understand a word she said, his little spirit now felt safe and accepted by her, and his body responded in health. That baby's face was healed in a very short time.

Many people's allergies develop as a result of not being loved properly by their parents. Over my thirty years of ministry, it has been my observation that some cases of eczema are due to inadequate touching and cuddling in infancy. In the case of the baby in New England, a lack of nurture and acceptance by his mother opened the door for the spirit of fear to affect him, even though he didn't understand what was happening to him. The key to his healing was the repentance of the parent to Father God for allowing an evil spirit of rejection to make the child feel unwanted. When the parent repented, the child was healed and nurtured at the spirit level first which then manifested in the healing of his skin/body.

We are on this journey to grow, to learn to sanctify ourselves in spirit, soul, and body. Prevent allergies by creating families that love and forgive one another. Teach them God's ways. Change may not happen overnight, but it will happen.

FEAR AS A BLOCK TO HEALING

One of the men involved with our ministry shared the experiences he had with fear and allergies in his household. Several years ago, when his daughter was not quite one year old, she developed seasonal allergies. She sneezed repeatedly, and her eyes were always filled with gunk. He was already working with Be in Health and was trying to understand and deal with the root cause of her allergic reactions. I asked him, "What are you doing about the allergies?" "We're giving her a children's antihistamine," he said, "and not letting her play outside until this season has passed. We've been thinking about tearing up our carpet."

Then I asked him, "Do you think it's possible that you are afraid of her reaction to the environment? That she senses your fear in the home, which is playing a role in her allergies?" Here, we have an example of the root being dealt with but there still being a block to the healing. The root was a fear in relationship, but the fear of the allergies themselves was a block. Do you see the difference?

He went home and talked it over with his wife. Together, they repented of that spirit of fear and cast down those fearful thoughts. Having repented and prayed for healing for their daughter, they decided not to worry and just let her be a child. One month later, their baby girl was healed of those allergies, and they have not returned to this day.

Remember that children can sense our insecurities and fears. As parents, we often try to protect our children out of love, but we can become the problem. Parents, a word to the wise! Don't hover over your children in fear regarding anything in their lives. If you act this way, you are teaching them to respond to the spirit of fear. Don't even hover over your older, unsaved children in fear. Get that spirit of fear away from them. Stand beside them in the faith of God instead!

INSIGHTS INTO ALLERGIES

Early in my journey of helping people, I received a phone call from a woman who was desperate. (I will refer to her as Margaret.) Margaret had spent ten years in near seclusion in a sanitary room with no carpeting and little furniture. Because of severe allergies, she had learned to avoid everything in her environment. She couldn't even spend time with or eat with her husband and children. She was down to eating only one or two foods each day.

Margaret explained that her medical diagnosis was Multiple Chemical Sensitivity/Environmental Illness (MCS/EI), which is a diagnosis given to someone who has an allergic reaction to many common chemicals in their environment, such as pesticides, perfumes, plastics, clothing, carpeting, and certain foods. There is a wide range of chronic symptoms, including headaches, muscle and joint pain, fatigue, rashes, asthma, memory loss, and confusion. Her doctors were convinced that the root of her allergies was exposure to pesticides that had completely destroyed her immune system.

Margaret explained her ailments, and then she pleaded with me, saying, "Oh, Pastor Wright, please come here to see me. I can't leave my room or fly on a plane. It will cost me my life." I was surprised by her request. Margaret lived on the other side of the country, and at that point, I had never traveled for the ministry. Quietly, I prayed, and then I responded, "Okay, Margaret. I don't know what I can do for you, but I will give you ten days of my life."

On the plane later that week, I opened my Bible to search for answers. James 1:5 tells us, *"If any of you lack wisdom, let him ask of God, that giveth to all men liberally, and upbraideth not; and it shall be given him."* So, I prayed and said to Father God. "Sir, this is a disease I know nothing about, and I'm going to minister to a stranger who I know nothing about. What am I doing? Have I lost my mind?" I searched the Scriptures to see if there was anything at all that was related to pesticides or environmental illnesses. Then, the Lord led me to Proverbs 17:22: *"A merry heart doeth good like a medicine: but a broken spirit drieth the bones."* As I meditated on that Scripture, I thought about the way God has created our bones. There is much more to them than what we usually think about—the hard skeleton that enables us to stand and move. In the center of our bones, there is a spongy material called the bone marrow that is continuously producing our red blood cells, white blood cells, and platelets. The white blood cells play a vital role in our immune system. God has created them to fight against invading bacteria, viruses, and fungi—to help destroy all harmful invaders in our bodies. We can't exist without a healthy immune system.

As I was meditating on Proverbs 17:22, *"...a broken spirit drieth the bones,"* I thought, "What could that mean, Lord? Could it mean a broken spirit, or a broken heart, dries up the soft tissue of the bone marrow, affects the white blood cells, and destroys the immune system?" God was revealing to me that a breakdown at the spiritual level can lead to a physiological breakdown in our bodies. This led me to wonder: "Lord, who broke this woman's heart?"

HEALING OF A BROKEN HEART

When I arrived to minister to this very ill woman, I tested out what I had read in Scripture. I asked, "Margaret, who has damaged you? Who was supposed to love you but didn't? Who has put this kind of dread or fear within you?" After a few quiet moments, she answered me, not with words but with tears.

I spent seven days of ministry with Margaret, helping her to understand Father God's love for her and challenging her to face fear in her life. No matter what had happened in her life, her relationship with Him was not broken. She repented of embracing the bitterness and unforgiveness that continually reminded her of painful hurts from the past. She repented of the fear that had brought her to a place of isolation while trying to protect herself from allergic reactions. The lie brought by Satan's kingdom led her to believe the world around her was killing her, but the true enemy was the spirit of fear, which caused her body to malfunction and deteriorate due to the fearful thoughts she meditated on day in and day out.

Margaret learned to recognize and cast down thoughts from Satan's kingdom—specifically, a fear of loving and being loved, which had driven her into isolation. She made the choice to trust God's Word over fearful thoughts of what could go wrong. Living a fearful, stressed-out life had led to her torment. But, remember, God's perfect love would destroy the fear in her life: *"There is no fear in love; but perfect love casteth out fear: because fear hath torment. He that feareth is not made perfect in love.* (1 John 4:18).

I explained to her what the fear and isolation had done to weaken her immune system. At the end of seven days of receiving the truth of God's Word, Margaret walked out of her room for the first time in years. She had no allergic reactions as she moved through the rooms in her home and sat with her husband and children at the table. Later that day, I went with her entire family to dinner at a steak restaurant called Sizzler. She was able to eat everything on that buffet! No allergic reactions. Margaret finally understood that she was loved by God, that He would protect her as He promised in His Word, and that she could love herself. Father God had healed her broken heart.

Let me add here that when you begin, in faith, to eat foods again that you have been allergic to, or if you begin to do this with your children, be sure to be led by God in the timing and how to proceed. Use wisdom, and, in many cases, make any changes carefully and incrementally.

WHAT IS A BROKEN HEART?

If we have a broken heart (or a broken spirit), we have been pierced, perhaps because of verbal, physical, or sexual abuse. As I mentioned earlier, being *pierced* happens when we feel the sting of abuse and sins against us. The enemy uses these tragedies to tempt us to become wounded and bitter, taking in the offense against us. Bitterness will tell us they "hurt" us, and we will dwell on their actions against us.

We may also embrace offenses against us and internalize them as self-hatred. Then, we become fearful in relationships in an attempt to protect ourselves from future hurts. If we allow those things to happen, the piercing will turn into a deep *wound* that does not heal. What we have in the end is a broken heart unless we repent to Father God for taking in the bitterness that hurt us.

These wounds go the very deepest because someone who was supposed to love us and take care of us has betrayed us. The truth of the matter is that we have all been accused, rejected, or treated poorly in the past. *Too often, we presume others should not sin against us.* We would like this to be true, but it is unrealistic. Can we truly expect imperfect people to love us *perfectly?* None of us is perfect. The truth of the matter is that we all have sinned and have fallen short of the glory of God. Remember the verse, *"all have sinned, and come short of the glory of God"* (Romans 3:23).

So, what should we do? Without question, we need to be willing to forgive others and turn to Father God and ask Him to convict us of sin in our own life. If we focus on our relationship to the Father, we can break patterns of sin and desolation in ourselves and in our family tree. It is only when someone stands up in their family line and stops blaming others for their problems that Father God may transform their life and provide a new path into the future for them and their generation. Even if we have ample evidence for why we have harbored resentment or anger, it will never lead us to a solution. It will only lead us to perpetuate the same cycles of sin that we have seen in our parents and grandparents. The psalmist prayed, *"Against thee, thee only, have I sinned, and done this evil in thy sight: that thou mightest be justified when thou speakest, and be clear when thou judgest"* (Psalm 51:4).

We understand that a broken heart does not allow a person to give and receive love without fear. They are filled with an intense fear that no one can be trusted and that they can never love or be loved by anyone again. That fear makes them guarded, and so they retreat into themselves, which leads to isolation. The person who suffers from a broken heart also believes that no one understands the pain they feel.

My doctorate is in Christian Therapeutic Counseling. I am not disengaged when I minister to people. When they grieve, I grieve with them. I have sat and wept with thousands of men and women whose hearts have been broken. So, if you are suffering from a broken heart, I know you from the inside out. You are trapped within your own self. You were never given a place to share your heart without shame and guilt. You have so much fear and even self-loathing because you were not loved properly.

ALLERGIES, HEALING, AND FOR MY LIFE

When I read in Proverbs 17:22 that a broken spirit dries up our bones, I realized the connection between thought and disease when it comes to people suffering from multiple allergies. That is when the Lord showed me that the common spiritual root of these multiple allergies, such as MCS/EI—and simple allergies, as well—is fear. In Margaret's case, the fear produced by her broken heart would not let her give or receive love in her relationships. At Be in Health, we have encountered many people who have MCS/EI who have suffered from emotional, verbal, or sexual abuse by a parent or someone else close to them. As a result, they are afraid to love without fear—and, remember, the Bible says in 1 John 4:18 that "*fear hath torment.*" Their tormented thought life of self-rejection and fear keeps them in bondage. Their freedom and healing come from repenting of these sins and embracing the truth in God's Word concerning the Father's love for them.

Recently, a woman named Kim attended one of our For My Life retreats. Kim had been diagnosed with MCS/EI and was down to eighty-one pounds. There were only three foods left that she could eat. Because she knew that she was dying, she had traveled to another state to visit her adult son one last time to say good-bye.

Thankfully, someone invited Kim to a For My Life retreat in Thomaston, Georgia, and she decided to search for healing one more time. During that week, Kim learned that God's perfect will is for health for His children. She repented of embracing the spirit of fear in her life, received God's truth for her, and began to gain her life back.

Over the next months, Kim embraced the path of freedom from disease. She walked out of Satan's kingdom by the Word of God, applying forgiveness, casting down fearful thoughts, and renewing her mind. Since then, she has gained fifty pounds and is healthy again. Kim and her husband now travel, enjoying life and God's creation together. She is another testament that the Father's love, and the power of His Word to heal, are always greater than the enemy's plan!

What has changed for thousands of people like Kim around the world who have been healed of their allergies after hearing these teachings? They have repented of following after sin and have chosen the Word of God instead. They are traveling on a day-by-day journey of discernment comparing their thoughts to the Word of God. When confronted with thoughts of fear, they choose to dwell on and follow the Word of God despite what they might feel. And they are free! *"Wherefore take unto you the whole armour of God, that ye may be able to withstand in the evil day, and having done all, to stand"* (Ephesians 6:13).

With time, our bodies will stop responding to the training of fear. Those who have been healed have observed their bodies no longer reacting to fear. The hypersensitivity and inflammation associated with allergies were healed. Their immune systems were healed, and their hearts were made whole. I am blessed that our team is being used by the Father to help others find release from chronic allergies.

In the coming days and weeks, you might find yourself being reminded of certain thoughts or issues that make you afraid. In those moments, don't shrink back! Go to Father God who loves you and repent for those spirits of fear so that you may be healed. Be encouraged. There is grace to help you in time of need!

Seeing then that we have a great high priest, that is passed into the heavens, Jesus the Son of God, let us hold fast our profession. For we have not an high priest which cannot be touched with the feeling of our infirmities; but was in all points tempted like as we are, yet without sin. Let us therefore come boldly unto the throne of grace, that we may obtain mercy, and find grace to help in time of need.

(Hebrews 4:14–16)

HEALING FOR BOTH MOTHER AND SON

MARIANNE

I went to à For My Life retreat seeking help for my son who had a terrible disease. I wasn't looking for help for myself, although I had suffered for years with celiac disease—which is a gluten allergy—and a shellfish allergy. None of the medical advice or alternative medicines had ever helped me.

While I was at the For My Life retreat, I realized that I had deep issues of fear and anxiety. I am the mother of eight children, and I know lots of things can go wrong in the world. Now that my son was sick, my fear was that I could lose him. I was so full of anxiety and fear that I couldn't sleep or eat.

I went to For My Life with an open heart. The first few days, I felt a movement within my stomach and intestines, and I felt like I was being healed. After being allergic to gluten for so long, I went to one of the leaders and said, "I think I am healed, but I'm afraid to eat the gluten." His counsel was to listen to God, and He would tell me when I should make the choice. That very day, I started to eat wheat products to see if I was really healed.

I couldn't believe it! No reaction! Before, I would have had a terrible headache by the next morning, with my eyes swollen shut.

It's so beautiful and amazing when God does something in your life! I'm so grateful. I'm filled with happiness, joy, and gratitude—overwhelming gratitude. My son was also restored to health through applying these biblical principles, and for that I am eternally grateful.

SEVEN

THE SPIRITUAL ROOTS OF
AUTOIMMUNE DISEASE

As you recall, I have recognized that 80 percent of problems with disease come from spiritual roots that are a result of a breakdown in our relationships: our relationship with God, His love, and His Word; our relationship with ourselves; or our relationship with others.

We have talked about how our relationship with God is restored through repentance, when we receive His forgiveness through Christ, cast down thoughts that are not from Him, and renew our minds by His Word. Our relationship with others is restored when we repent, when we forgive them or ask for their forgiveness, and when we cast aside hatred and malice. But what about the breakdown in relationship with ourselves? Do you know how many people struggle with self-hatred, self-rejection, and a belief that they are unlovable? Do you know how many people do not know how to love themselves?

Is there a scriptural foundation for loving ourselves? Actually, there is clear evidence from Scripture, in both the Old and the New Testament, that we are to love ourselves. Leviticus 19:18 says, *"Thou shalt not avenge, nor bear any grudge against the children of thy people, but thou shalt love thy neighbour as thyself: I am the LORD."* And we read in Ephesians 5:28, *"So ought men to love their wives as their own bodies. He that loveth his wife loveth himself."*

If I find a man who is unkind to his wife or who cannot be affectionate toward her, I know that man does not love himself. Additionally, people who are hard on themselves and have a hard time letting go of their own failures and past sins have a difficult time forgiving other people, as well. Their tendency to be hard on themselves leads to harshness toward others.

I have coined a term that we use in the For My Life retreat. It is the "unloving" spirit. What does it mean to be "unloving"? To understand this, we need to consider what love is according to Scripture. There are many definitions in the world of love, but the term *love*, or *charity*, is clearly defined in 1 Corinthians, chapter 13.

Charity suffereth long, and is kind; charity envieth not; charity vaunteth not itself, is not puffed up, doth not behave itself unseemly, seeketh not her own, is not easily provoked, thinketh no evil; rejoiceth not in iniquity, but rejoiceth in the truth; beareth all things, believeth all things, hopeth all things, endureth all things. (1 Corinthians 13:4–7)

True love is not selfish. It does not harbor grudges; it is not self-defensive, protecting itself from being hurt by others; and it is not self-seeking. Love is self-less. On the other hand, unloving spirits as I describe them are quite the opposite; they are the kingdom of self. Self-hatred, self-accusation, and self-rejection are obvious examples.

My definition of an unloving spirit is the inability to give or receive love without fear. Remember, according to Scripture, it is perfect love that casts out fear. Therefore, if someone is unable to receive love, they are afraid and bound by a spirit of fear. The best example I can give of someone with an unloving spirit is a person who cannot receive a hug. Have you ever met someone like that? When you go to hug them, it's like hugging a telephone pole. Their arms and back become stiff because they cannot receive the hug. This rigidity is evidence of fear.

The core problem here does not originate with humans. It is first a spiritual problem between each of us individually and Father God. If we refuse to believe that Father God loves us, we will never fulfill our mission as humans. There are many people searching for "self-love," but it is based upon comparisons or standards of performance and accomplishment.

If we judge ourselves by metrics of performance, then an infant would have little to no value and an elderly person would be considered less important. It is the reason many humans struggle with their value. They determine value by superficial standards. Then what should be our standard? In God's eyes, we have equal value regardless of accomplishment. Our value originates with Father God. He loved us before we knew Him. It begins and ends with Him. We have value not because of our accomplishments but because our Creator made us and sees us as valuable to Him, and that is the end of the conversation. *"We love him, because he first loved us"* (1 John 4:19).

If God says it, He means it, and it is a closed subject. Is there anyone in creation with a greater position than Father God? No. Therefore, if God be for us, who can be against us? As the apostle Paul put it, *"What shall we then say to these things? If God be for us, who can be against us?"* (Romans 8:31).

ARE WE ALLERGIC TO OURSELVES?

So, how does self-hatred—what I call an unloving spirit—negatively affect the immune system? A person who struggles with self-hatred has believed thoughts from Satan's kingdom about themselves. These thoughts tell them they never measure up and constantly remind them of past failures to reinforce their negative self-image. Remember from our earlier teaching that if we do not reject or cast down these thoughts, the hypothalamus responds to the temptation, triggering the body to respond as if something is seriously wrong. The hypothalamus begins to misfire and sends the wrong impulses to other parts of the endocrine system. The result is that the immune system will weaken and become compromised as the body physically attacks itself. In an autoimmune response, the body is literally treating *its own tissue* as a foreign invader because the person believes they are the problem.

The bottom line of this malfunction? Autoimmune disease. The body becomes allergic to itself! How can this be? Because the person has become allergic to themselves spiritually. Satan's kingdom has persuaded them that they are their own worst enemy. As a result, the immune system is compromised, and the white corpuscles mistakenly identify the antigen markers on the healthy cells in the body as a disease or an invader and attacks them. The white corpuscles, or T cells, receive the signal that the healthy tissue is the enemy, and they will either destroy it or produce inflammation in a particular area. An autoimmune blood test will show that antibodies are attacking their own healthy tissue.

The body attacks itself because the person is attacking themselves spiritually in self- rejection, self-hatred, and self-bitterness. There is a spiritual dynamic that comes into play in which the white corpuscles are redirected to attack living tissue while ignoring the true enemies, or invaders, which include bacteria, viruses, and cancers. As the person continues to attack himself or herself spiritually by self-rejection and self-loathing, the body finally agrees, and the white corpuscles start attacking the body itself. Quit making yourself the enemy and being allergic to yourself! That is a high price to pay for not loving yourself.

AN UNLOVING SPIRIT

From my years of ministry, I have concluded that most autoimmune diseases are the result of an unloving spirit that produces feelings of not being loved and not feeling accepted. This leads to self-rejection, self-hatred, and self-bitterness, coupled with guilt. In fact, it could be said that autoimmune diseases are primarily a self-hatred disease with a spirit of fear (producing anxiety and stress) attached to it. Anxiety and stress are a direct biological outcome of rejecting who God's Word says you are and choosing to believe evil thoughts from the enemy instead. To accept yourself, you need to make the decision to trust what Father God has said about you. If He says you are fearfully and wonderfully made, then what are you? Fearfully and wonderfully made! *"I will praise thee; for I am fearfully and wonderfully made: marvellous are thy works; and that my soul knoweth right well"* (Psalm 139:14).

You cannot talk or reason yourself into believing the Word of God. If you cannot believe what the Bible has said, then there is an "anti-Christ," or evil, spirit against Christ that is blocking you from believing it. *"And every spirit that confesseth not that Jesus Christ is come in the flesh is not of God: and this is that spirit of antichrist, whereof ye have heard that it should come; and even now already is it in the world"* (1 John 4:3).

Calling the unloving spirit an anti-Christ spirit can confuse people because they believe I am talking about the end-times figure known as the "Antichrist." In His preincarnate form, Jesus was God the Word. So these spirits are *against* or *anti*-Christ because they oppose His Word and His mission when He came to earth as a human.

In the beginning was the Word, and the Word was with God, and the Word was God. The same was in the beginning with God. All things were made by him; and without him was not any thing made that was made....And the Word was made flesh, and dwelt among us, (and we beheld his glory, the glory as of the only begotten of the Father,) full of grace and truth. (John 1:1–3, 14)

If you say that God does not love you or that you are unlovable, that is the work of an anti-Christ spirit. Have you considered that when you say you are unlovable, you are in rebellion and opposition against the Word of God? There are plenty of Scriptures that plainly state that Father God loves you. In fact, the very reason Jesus was sent to earth and died on the cross was because of the love Father God has for you. *"For God so loved the world, that he gave his only begotten Son, that whosoever believeth in him should not perish, but have everlasting life"* (John 3:16).

When you argue with the Word of God that He has accepted you, then an evil spirit of self-rejection has joined you. It will oppose *all* Scriptures that reinforce God's love for and acceptance of you. That spirit will torment you until you repent to Father God for believing self-rejection instead of believing the Word of God, which tells you that because of His grace you are accepted in the beloved: *"To the praise of the glory of his grace, wherein he hath made us accepted in the beloved"* (Ephesians 1:6).

Self-rejection leads to being bound by sin that will not let you accept God's righteousness for you. You can't believe the promises of redemption and freedom from God in His Word. You think they only apply to others. The result is that the spirit-soul-body connection is in play and the body attacks itself. Autoimmune disease is the consequence.

There are approximately a hundred autoimmune diseases or disorders. They include diabetes 1, Graves' disease, lupus, Crohn's disease, psoriasis, rheumatoid arthritis, multiple sclerosis, and so many more. The medical community has no idea what to do with autoimmune disease. Doctors don't understand the spiritual roots of disease, so they manage you in your sin. Not only does the cause elude them, but they also consider all autoimmune diseases to be incurable. Thankfully, the word *incurable* is not in the Bible! We have seen tremendous results through For My Life in the healing of autoimmune diseases when people have embraced the truth of these teachings.

WHAT IS SELF-HATRED?

We shared earlier that self-hatred is devastating because it makes you a god unto yourself. How do you become a god unto yourself? By exalting Satan's lies over the Word of God. If Father God has said you have value, and you reject His Word, you have put yourself in the position of "god" over your own life. This may sound bizarre, since we are talking about hating yourself, but if you reject what God has said, you have made yourself greater than the Word of God.

How does self-hatred take hold in your life? It often begins with the accusations of others toward you, specifically authority figures such as grandparents, parents, teachers, and even peers. In many cases, self-hatred begins with unmet expectations of acceptance and approval. If we are routinely told that we do not measure up or that we are not acceptable, we are set up to receive self-hatred. At some point, we may accept that these words are true, begin to believe them about ourselves, and internalize them toward ourselves.

The Bible does not explicitly say we need to "forgive ourselves." In fact, there are many people who teach similar concepts outside the church. When we say we need to forgive ourselves in a scriptural sense, it may need some explanation. If we fail or make a mistake, self-hatred will continually remind us of these failures and why we cannot live them down. Many people who struggle with self-hatred are extremely hard on themselves and beat themselves up when they fail to meet their own expectations of themselves.

What we must do instead is acknowledge self-hatred as an evil spirit. It is not just a psychological state. In order to overcome self-hatred, we need to repent to Father God of embracing the expectations of others concerning us and for allowing this evil spirit to beat us up over our failures. Forgiving ourselves requires repenting of agreeing with self-hatred and letting go of what it says about us and taking hold of the forgiveness Father God has given us by faith. Remember 1 John 1:9, which says, *"If we confess our sins, he is faithful and just to forgive us our sins, and to cleanse us from all unrighteousness."*

The truth is, you will make mistakes and fail in your journey as a believer. You must be willing to get up when you fall. What defines the difference between the just man and the wicked man is not failure but a willingness to get back up and repent when he falls in failure. As it says in Proverbs 24:16, *"For a just man falleth seven times, and riseth up again: but the wicked shall fall into mischief."*

You are not rejected by God, so why are you rejecting yourself? When you hate yourself, it results in self-resentment, self-bitterness, and self-unforgiveness. God forgives you, but you may not believe you deserve forgiveness, so you won't forgive yourself. Do you realize that you are rejecting Jesus's work for you on the cross? You are telling Him that His death was insufficient to free you from who you are or what you have done wrong.

This is a really important issue concerning our need to be loved. We all need to be loved. God loves you, but something has gotten in between you and God, so that you don't feel loved—you feel rejected. That is when you become allergic to yourself. You may have an identity in the world—it might even be a successful identity—but you don't have an identity in God. God is the author and sustainer of all that He has made, including you. You must find and accept your identity in Him.

Yea doubtless, and I count all things but loss for the excellency of the knowledge of Christ Jesus my Lord: for whom I have suffered the loss of all things, and do count them but dung, that I may win Christ, and be

found in him, not having mine own righteousness, which is of the law,
but that which is through the faith of Christ, the righteousness which is
of God by faith.   (Philippians 3:8–9)

UNCOVERING SPECIFIC AUTOIMMUNE DISEASES

Let's consider some specific autoimmune diseases and how an incorrect spirituality can negatively affect the spirit, soul, and body.

TYPE 1 DIABETES AND REJECTION

Spiritual:

A spirit of rejection joins a person because of the rejection of a father.

Soul/Thoughts:

Although adults can still develop diabetes 1, it usually starts in childhood and is a direct result of living in a hostile or unloving family environment, particularly with rejection from a father. The child begins to think, "Something is wrong with me." They attack themselves in their minds and with their mouths; the result is that the body attacks the body.

Body/Physical:

Type 1 diabetes is an autoimmune disease in which the pancreas no longer produces the insulin needed to control sugar in the body. The body's own immune system—which was created to fight harmful bacteria and viruses—mistakenly destroys the insulin-producing islet cells in the pancreas. The white corpuscles mistakenly identify the antigen markers on the pancreatic islets and attack and "eat" them. As a result, the pancreas no longer produces the insulin needed to move sugar (glucose) into the cells, and the sugar builds up in the bloodstream. This can lead to life-threatening conditions.

LUPUS AND GUILT

Spiritual:

With lupus, the primary trigger point or spiritual root is an evil spirit of guilt.

Soul/Thoughts:

Because of some unresolved matter in their life, the person refuses to forgive themselves and carries guilt. Since they are unable to forgive themselves, they are tormented with thoughts stemming from the inability to receive freedom from past perceived or real failures.

Body/Physical:

Lupus is an autoimmune disease in which the white corpuscles mistakenly target the antigen markers on the connective tissue of the organs. Therefore, once again, the immune system attacks the body it was supposed to protect. Our organs are the core of our biology. So, as the white corpuscles begin to destroy the connective tissue around the organs, the person experiences pain, fatigue, fever, shortness of breath, and other symptoms.

Specific Insights:

Guilt is a powerful force against us. It is essential for us to understand Satan's devices and forgive ourselves. Guilt defies a risen Christ and forgiveness. Guilt is an anti-Christ spirit. Guilt doesn't come from God! Why hang on to things in your personality that don't come from God?

Lupus is considered incurable, but through years of ministry, we have been blessed to see many people healed of the disease. A few years ago, I ministered to one woman who had an extreme case of lupus. She had also had multiple miscarriages. When the white corpuscles were eating the connective tissue, it was very painful and created inflammation throughout her body, including on the umbilical cord materials. The woman had been experiencing guilt even before the miscarriages began, but her guilt increased, even though the miscarriages were not her fault.

Once she was released from the spirit of guilt and embraced the truth of God's love for her, she was healed of lupus. Shortly afterward, she became pregnant and carried her first child to full term. She was saved and converted in her thinking, her personality changed, and she received the gift of health on this earth, a restored relationship with herself, and a restored relationship with her God!

RHEUMATOID ARTHRITIS AND SELF-HATRED

Spiritual:

Anything that relates to the skeleton or bones has an identity problem as its spiritual root, such as comparing ourselves to others. Many people with rheumatoid arthritis suffer from self-accusation.

Soul/Thoughts:

They don't accept themselves as they are. They think something about them is inferior. They have a very negative way of viewing themselves, the world, and God. As a result, they become allergic to themselves. We need to understand that we are meant to be unique individuals and not clones of anyone else. We are fearfully and wonderfully made. We are not made in the image of another human being—we are made in the image of God.

The saddest part of rheumatoid arthritis is that the person believes they are not as good as everyone else. Then, as their joints lose flexibility, parts of their body become deformed, with misshapen fingers and bent legs. In the end, the individual looks worse and feels worse about themselves. It is crucial that they repent of their negative self-projections and begin to find their identity according to the Word of God.

Body/Physical:

Rheumatoid arthritis is a disfiguring autoimmune disease. Once again, the white corpuscles are influenced by a spirit and misidentify the antigen markers on the connective cartilage of the joints. They say to that cartilage, "Wow, you're the enemy!" The white corpuscles attack the body by destroying its connective cartilage, and inflammation occurs.

MULTIPLE SCLEROSIS AND IDENTITY REJECTION

Spiritual:

I need to be very frank here and say that multiple sclerosis is deeply rooted in self-hatred.

Soul/Thoughts:

The person questions, "Why am I here?" "Who am I?" and "Who cares?" This goes beyond an identity issue to the total rejection of one's identity rooted in self-hatred.

Body/Physical:

Multiple sclerosis (MS) is an autoimmune disease that affects the nervous system. In the case of MS, the immune system malfunctions, and the white corpuscles destroy the fatty substance that coats and protects nerve fibers in the brain and spinal cord. This coating over our nerves is called the myelin sheath.

The best way to describe the myelin sheath is to compare it to the insulation coating on electrical wires. You have a copper wire that is transmitting the electricity. That wire is covered with insulation to protect people from being shocked and to protect the wire from being destroyed. Our nerves are created in a similar way. We have a myelin sheath encasing every nerve to protect us from nerve pain and to protect the nerves from damage.

With multiple sclerosis, the white corpuscles mistakenly recognize an antigen marker for disease on the myelin sheath. As the white corpuscles take a bite out of the myelin sheath, that's called a sclerosis. Multiple sclerosis means multiple bites of the myelin sheath around multiple nerves. The white corpuscles can sever the nerve itself once they destroy the myelin sheath, and nerve damage can become progressively worse. In some cases, the limbs lose activity.

Specific Insights:

I did a conference a couple of years ago called "Who Am I?" in which I discussed those three very important questions: "Who am I?" "Why am I here?" "Who cares?" These are the battles I see even with Christians. We have an orphan's mentality. Who cares? The Father cares! Your acceptance of His love can defeat autoimmune disorders in your life.

A disease of self-rejection results when you do not accept who you are in creation. Guilt and shame follow you. You're always looking over your shoulder for somebody else's approval and not getting it. Some of you are living in families that do not know how to love each other. Others have families that are like Job's friends. They act like they are there for you, but they're really accusing you. But you have a Father. You have *the* Father. Don't embrace the principles of death. Stop it. Embrace the principles of life.

Remind yourself, "I may have a disease, but I am not a disease!" Don't call it "my disease." There is sin that has been tormenting you, but you are not the sin. You are a child of God! Accept the Father's great love for you; He has called you to be His own! As it says in Jeremiah 31:3, *"The LORD hath appeared of old unto me, saying, Yea, I have loved thee with an everlasting love: therefore with lovingkindness have I drawn thee."*

CROHN'S DISEASE AND PERFORMANCE DISORDERS

Spiritual:

It's a constant, constant, constant self-conflict issue surrounding performance. This means there is a spirit of fear driving a person to perform, and there is an evil spirit of self-conflict that also requires repentance.

Soul/Thoughts:

The person with Crohn's disease can hyperventilate in fear that there might be a problem going on, even when there is no problem.

Body/Physical:

Crohn's disease is an autoimmune disease where the neurotransmitters are once again giving a false signal to the white corpuscles. The white corpuscles decide that the antigen marker for an invader is on the lining of the intestines. As they begin to "eat" the intestinal lining, it produces inflammation, ulceration, bleeding, and pain.

Specific Insights:

In studying case history after case history, I have concluded that Crohn's is a performance disorder in which the individual is extremely driven to do everything right in order to keep the people around them happy. There is guilt involved with Crohn's disease, as well, because the person doesn't believe they actually do anything right. As a result, the patient becomes a false burden bearer of others. They pick up other people's issues and blame themselves if things don't go right for these others. They blame themselves for other people's unhappiness, as if they were responsible for other people's failures as well as their own.

GRAVES' DISEASE AND THE THYROID

Spiritual:

The spiritual root behind Graves' disease is a performance disorder similar to that causing Crohn's disease. A person takes on the burdens of others, and this leads to self-accusation and guilt.

Soul/Thoughts:

Someone with Graves' disease feels responsible for others as though they had failed them when they do not make the decisions that you believe are right for their lives. The truth is, you are not responsible for the decisions of other people. You cannot control their journey, whether they do what is right or wrong before God, and you are not at fault despite their accusations against you.

Body/Physical:

Graves' disease is an autoimmune disease in which the white corpuscles congregate together in the thyroid. This produces a swelling that causes the thyroid to overproduce the hormone thyroxin. This condition is also referred to as hyperthyroidism. With Graves' disease, the individual experiences excessive fatigue, heart palpitations, a developing goiter, and bulging eyes. Graves' disease usually appears in females and, if left untreated, can be life-threatening.

Specific Insights:

Medical science's answer to Graves' disease is to use radioactive chemicals to destroy the thyroid, and then to put the patient on thyroid medicine for the rest of their life. God's prescription is that the person be healed of the underlying roots that are causing the disease.

There is a woman in ministry whom my wife, Donna, and I know very well; I will call her Jeanine. A few years ago, Jeanine called me from California worried about a medical diagnosis concerning her thyroid. Her doctor told her, "You have Graves' disease. I need to destroy your thyroid with radioactive iodine so that we can defeat the disease."

Now, Jeanine is not only a strong, well-grounded Christian, but she has been around our Be in Health teachings for several years. Feeling uncertain about the procedure, she called me and said, "I have a well-respected doctor who is also a member of my church. He has diagnosed me with Graves' disease. I already have the beginning of a goiter and bulging in my eyes. The disease is progressive, so the doctor wants to destroy my thyroid in order to cure it. What do you think?"

First, I asked her, "Did God give you a thyroid in creation?"

"Yes," she responded.

"Okay," I continued, "I know a little bit about autoimmune diseases, and I know about you. Jeanine, you just care too much. You have a performance disorder.

"You've got all these people coming to your house; you teach them, and you try to get them well. They won't listen to you. They won't do the first principles, but they keep coming back, and you are taking on their failures as though they were your own. Admit it; they are wearing you out. You feel responsible for them, and now you feel like you have failed them."

She began to cry. "You just know me too well," she told me.

"Jeanine, you have embraced guilt and self-accusation," I said. "You need to repent to God." Then I asked her, "Do you know that if your doctor destroys your thyroid, you will get another thyroid disease called Hashimoto's disease? You're going to exchange one disease for another. It's all you're going to get!"

Jeanine knew that I had done extensive research on many diseases, including Graves' disease. Yes, one procedure is the use of radioactive iodine, but another procedure includes a drug that you can take that will stop the forward progress of Graves' disease instantly, as long as you keep taking the medication. Jeanine was already in an advanced stage of Graves' disease, but she was just learning the truth about the spiritual roots of the disease. We needed to buy some time so that she could apply these scriptural truths to her life and begin her healing process. So, I suggested, "Go back to your doctor and ask him if there is a drug you can take to stop the forward progress of this disease."

She did it, and began by saying to him, "Doctor, I've been talking to Pastor Henry Wright."

He retorted, "What's a pastor know about my industry?"

She didn't respond to that but only continued, "Dr. Wright said there's a drug I can take that would stop the progress of the disease, and here's the name of the drug. Did he tell me the truth?"

The doctor responded, "Yes, he told you the truth. But if we just get rid of your thyroid, you won't have to take the drug."

She asked, "Will I get Hashimoto's disease as an exchange?"

"Yes, but at least you'll be alive."

"I want the drug," she told him with resolve. "Please prescribe it. I've got some work to do on my sanctification."

Jeanine began to go to God to change her heart and mind, confessing her sins of taking on the burdens of other people's lives. She prayed and began to meditate on the Word daily from a sincere heart. She took those thoughts of guilt and self-accusation captive to the obedience of Jesus Christ, casting them down because they were not from God but from the enemy. All the while, she was on this medication.

About a month later, Jeanine started having weird symptoms and reactions. She went back to the doctor and told him, "For the last month that I've been taking this medication, I've been feeling worse and worse."

"Let me do a test," he answered. When he came back a short time later, the doctor was smiling broadly. "Jeanine, you are reacting to the medication," he admitted.

"Why?" she asked.

"Because your thyroid is functioning normally!" he announced. "There are no more signs of Graves' disease!"

Praise God! All autoimmune disease activity had stopped. God had healed Jeanine's thyroid. Within a short time, the bulging eyes and the goiter went away. This woman, my friend, is alive and well today with a healthy thyroid because she applied God's truth.

One side note: Hashimoto's is a different autoimmune disease in which the thyroid is being destroyed by the immune system, resulting in an underproduction of the hormone thyroxine. As a result, many of the body's functions slow down. Weight gain and fatigue are common. These symptoms are treated by thyroid medicines to increase the level of thyroxine. Hashimoto's is also deeply rooted in self-accusation.

Are you learning anything? Is disease happenstance, or is it a planned event? I think you can see that the enemy is smarter than you realized. The devil is banking on your ignorance. He expects you to be ruled by your feelings and emotions and not by the Word of God. But God is greater than anything the enemy can send your way, if you will trust Him and His Word of truth.

THE ANTIDOTE TO AUTOIMMUNE DISEASE

I have the antidote to self-hatred and to autoimmune disorders. No doctor can give this prescription to you. It is Psalm 139. Read it. Read all of it. Read it over and over and over again until you embrace its truth from your heart. You will find yourself and how God thinks about you in Psalm 139. Below is just a portion of it:

For thou hast possessed my reins: thou hast covered me in my mother's womb. I will praise thee; for I am fearfully and wonderfully made: marvellous are thy works; and that my soul knoweth right well. My substance was not hid from thee, when I was made in secret, and curiously wrought in the lowest parts of the earth. Thine eyes did see my substance, yet being unperfect; and in thy book all my members were written, which in continuance were fashioned, when as yet there was none of them. How precious also are thy thoughts unto me, O God! how great is the sum of them! If I should count them, they are more in number than the sand: when I awake, I am still with thee.

(Psalm 139:13–18)

Embrace the truth of Psalm 139 that you are *"fearfully and wonderfully made"* and that God's thoughts toward you are *"precious"* and *"more in number than the sand"*! Repent of hating and rejecting yourself to this God who loves you. Stop this self-accusation. Quit arguing that point with God. You do not have to suffer self-accusation any longer! If you will believe God's

Word, you will be set free! Remember, the enemy is the accuser of the brethren! Why would you believe the enemy instead of believing the living God and what He says in Psalm 139? Satan poisoned you. I'm giving you the antidote. I'm giving you the Word of God so that you will be delivered and healed!

God sent His Holy Spirit specially to gather you to Himself through Jesus's atonement, and you responded, "Yes." Now you need to embrace that message of salvation and what it means for you each and every day. When you were born again, you became a son or daughter of the Father of all spirits. Why would you doubt Him now? *"What shall we then say to these things? If God be for us, who can be against us?"* (Romans 8:31).

Let God be true in your life! I don't care what your mother or father said to you. I don't care if you were put up for adoption. I don't care if you were an orphan. You're not an orphan anymore! God has adopted you as His own! *"For ye have not received the spirit of bondage again to fear; but ye have received the Spirit of adoption, whereby we cry, Abba, Father"* (Romans 8:15).

Are you ready to be purified like gold? Are you ready to have the dross burned out of you, the stuff that's not of God? Are you really ready to change? I'm after you to help you. I am writing this to create a revelation of thought that will lead you to take ownership of your life. I didn't study this subject for decades just to give you some knowledge. I want you to grasp the truth that you don't have to be sick. Based on the promises of God, you can decide to have life and to have it more abundantly. (See John 10:10.) But it depends on your awakening to the kingdom of God and His ways. I'm after you because the Lord is after you with His truth. I'm just happy to serve Him for your benefit.

HEALED OF PARKINSON'S DISEASE

BILL

Bill was one of our For My Life retreat participants a few years ago, and he was suffering from Parkinson's disease. Here he shares his testimony of complete healing.

When my father was eighty years old, he was in a wheelchair and died of advanced Parkinson's disease. My older brother was also in a wheelchair and died at eighty-one of advanced Parkinson's disease. When I hit my seventies, I was diagnosed with the early stages of Parkinson's. The doctor said it was a family disease and there was nothing he could do for me.

Well, I wouldn't accept that. I had read Dr. Wright's first book, *A More Excellent Way*, and discovered that the spiritual roots of Parkinson's were spirits of unresolved rejection, abandonment, and deferred hope. When I attended the For My Life retreat, I repented of allowing those spirits to reign in my heart and mind. I told those evil spirits to leave me and never return.

For the next six months, I renewed my mind; I read and meditated on every Scripture about hope that I found in the Bible.

At the end of that time, I went to a follow-up visit with my endocrinologist. After he examined me, he said, "Bill, you don't have Parkinson's disease any longer. It wasn't anything I did. Stop your medication. I don't need to see you again!"

Praise God! I am healed! I am well! I am a miracle!

EIGHT

THE SPIRITUAL ROOTS OF CARDIOVASCULAR DISEASE

The conventional methods for preventing cardiovascular disease primarily focus on nutrition and exercise. I have been convicted by the Lord of the need to practice something called moderation—or, as some translations of the Bible call it, self-control—when it comes to certain foods.

Our body is a temple of the Holy Spirit, and we shouldn't be abusing it with too much food or the wrong kind of food. I had to learn to be moderate in my eating habits. Food is enjoyable—preparing it and eating it! In the past, I worked professionally as a chef in several restaurants, and I have always loved to cook at home. It's an art form to me.

Formerly, with my favorite foods, I found it difficult to eat in moderation. With barbecued ribs, two slabs were never enough. Now, when we go out for barbecue, having just two bones is perfect. I eat what I like, but I don't overindulge. It is fun learning self-control, and it has helped my health, enabling me to lose nearly eighty pounds in the last few years. (However, I have to admit that I have always struggled a bit with Krispy Kreme doughnuts!)

NUTRITION WON'T REPLACE RIGHTEOUSNESS

Now, even though body maintenance is important, we need to look at what else the Word of God has to say about food: *"For the kingdom of God is not meat and drink; but righteousness, and peace, and joy in the Holy Ghost"* (Romans 14:17).

It's good for us to eat balanced meals of nutritional foods that can replace what the body has used up in homeostasis, but if you think nutrition is the only basis for health and longevity, you are wrong. If you have anger, stress, rage, and fear trapped inside of you, destroying your body's ability to fight off disease, then nutrition cannot entirely prevent heart disease from coming your way.

Nutrition is important, but it does not replace our need for righteousness, peace, and joy in the Holy Spirit.

EXERCISE IN GODLINESS

Moderate exercise can strengthen our bodies and our minds, but exercise isn't the total solution to our health either. We know people who got plenty of exercise but died because of a spiritual root that destroyed their immune system or damaged their heart. Some individuals who have attended For My Life with heart-related illnesses have maintained strict dietary and exercise routines for years and still developed cardiovascular issues. It is important to point out that, according to Scripture, exercise profits little: *"For bodily exercise profiteth little: but godliness is profitable unto all things, having promise of the life that now is, and of that which is to come"* (1 Timothy 4:8).

Why does Scripture say that exercise "profits little"? It is not because exercise is useless but because godliness is profitable both in this life and for eternity. The last time I checked, bodily exercise does not lead to eternal salvation. God is assuring us that exercising godliness will help in this life—with our health—and in the life to come.

MY PERSONAL JOURNEY

There are spiritual issues that are of central importance to this conversation so that we can have good health, both physically *and* spiritually. I have had my own journey around cardiovascular illness, related to both physical and spiritual issues. I am not perfect. There is the impression that because I have dedicated my life to understanding the spiritual roots of disease, I must never get sick. Many people were shocked when I had a life-threatening heart attack years ago. Was that evidence that these principles do not work? No. It was evidence that I am an imperfect human, and I am not sinless.

In 2011, I was conducting a For My Life conference in the city of Port of Spain, Trinidad and Tobago. Just a half hour into the first night of the conference, I began to sweat profusely and feel ill. I was rushed to the hospital. Within twenty-four hours, my wife, Donna, arrived from the States. I'd had a massive heart attack, and my heart was severely damaged. I would need triple bypass surgery to have a chance at survival. The doctor's prognosis: I probably wouldn't make it through the surgery. Thankfully, Father God had other plans for my life.

The heart attack and its aftermath have been quite a journey. At first, the doctors were treating me as if my death was imminent. They believed that their only job was to keep me alive long enough to fly me home to the United States. But with God's faithfulness, I made it through the surgery.

In the days ahead, it was still not clear to the medical community whether I would make it or not. I wish I could say that I was healed soon after, but there was serious damage done to my physical heart. Yet, despite the doubt and concerns of my doctors, I had to make a choice to believe the Word of God, even while cooperating with the medical team. Again, my statement is genuine—I am not against the medical community. I have had surgeries and taken medication because of these heart issues, and I appreciate that these medical interventions have helped to keep me alive. At the same time, I trust Father God as the One who ultimately sustains life.

I chose not to become hopeless because of a medical prognosis. I made the firm decision to hold on to the Word of God and His promises for my life and my health, daily taking "Gos-pills" from God's Word—Scriptures such as the following—to move me toward healing:

Then he said unto them, Go your way, eat the fat, and drink the sweet, and send portions unto them for whom nothing is prepared: for this day is holy unto our LORD: neither be ye sorry; for the joy of the LORD is your strength. (Nehemiah 8:10)

A merry heart doeth good like a medicine: but a broken spirit drieth the bones.

(Proverbs 17:22)

I shall not die, but live, and declare the works of the Lord.

(Psalm 118:17)

It is by these principles that God has led me throughout my journey as a believer. Because of Jesus's provision through the cross, I began walking out my faith in this situation, following hope and faith, not fear. I have long outlived the initial prognosis made after the heart attack. If I had embraced hopelessness and despair, I would have had no faith, and I probably would have died years ago. Instead, I embraced what I had been teaching others and became a happy, agreeable patient! In fact, when the doctors in Trinidad and Tobago gave me the letter of referral to a doctor in the States, they wrote, "Let us refer to you this most pleasant pastor from Georgia." My being called a pleasant pastor was a miracle in itself!

In the past, I "thundered" when I spoke. I could become very animated and loud because I was fighting for people's spiritual freedom. I wanted humanity to understand all the benefits Father God has for them. After the heart attack, my presentation softened and my demeanor changed, but my desire to care for others remained steadfast. I like to say, "I'm a work in progress. Excuse my dust!" What does that mean? It means I might say and do things the wrong way, or even say something that offends you. Are you willing to forgive me for these shortcomings? Are we all willing to forgive one another when we fail each other in relationship?

My journey of ministering to others was not born out of a desire to become an expert. It was and has always been because of the love Father God placed in my heart for humanity. Are you okay with the fact that the one writing to you is "just a guy"? When I started praying for and teaching people, God was the One who healed them, and He is still the Healer. I just showed up with a heartfelt willingness to pray for others. I am not a "spiritual superstar." There is only one "Superstar," and He (Jesus) is sitting or standing at the right hand of the Father. God calls flawed humans to represent Him. I am one of them, and so are you. It's okay that we are on a journey toward health and healing.

It is tragic to realize the unrealistic standards we set for humans. God does not call people to serve Him because they are perfect. He calls them because He has chosen them for His purposes. If you see someone in a leadership position who has flaws and problems, it is important to understand that Father God sees those issues, too, but that does not stop Him from calling a person to a position of leadership. The problem is idolatry. Too many people are looking for a human to be a "god" to them. I am not your god. I am a servant of Father God serving you with truth from the Bible. Will you allow me, your brother, to minister truth to you, even when I am on a journey of sanctification? One of the most precious moments I remember seeing was a person in a wheelchair ministering to another person in a wheelchair. We cannot wait for a "spiritual superstar" to show up. We need to be willing to serve and care for one another.

Confess your faults to one another, and pray for one another, that ye may be healed. The effectual fervent prayer of a righteous man availeth much.   (James 5:16)

LOVE AND OUR HEART

After the heart attack, I personally observed the principles that God uses to strengthen and restore our bodies. Shortly after I arrived back home from Trinidad and Tobago, I experienced congestive heart failure— irregular heartbeats, shortness of breath, coughing, dizziness, and fatigue. When I went to the heart clinic in Atlanta, I could not walk twenty feet without collapsing. They had to roll me into the clinic in a wheelchair. A year later, I walked back into that clinic. The cardiologist did a double take and said, "Whoa, Henry, is that you?" "Yes, it's me," I said with a smile. God's Word was at work in my body and my life.

During a medical checkup months later, my cardiologist exclaimed, "Henry, I don't know why you're here; I have nothing to offer you. I have no suggestions. You're supposed to either be dead or be wheeled in here on a stretcher half asleep. Yet, here you are, vital and alert. I don't know what to do with you. I'll see you in six months."

As a result of the heart attack, I developed secondary kidney issues and had to see a nephrologist, a doctor who specializes in kidney health as it relates to the heart. After watching my journey, the doctor told my wife, Donna, and me, "I attribute your remarkable recovery from a death disease to three things, none of which has to do with medicine or my work with you. All I do is monitor your progress.

"These are the three things," she continued. "Number one, your incredible belief in God." I didn't know she had noticed that much. "Number two, who you are on the inside." Remember, the Bible says, *"As he thinketh in his heart, so is he"* (Proverbs 23:7). The Bible also says, *"The spirit of a man will sustain his infirmity; but a wounded spirit who can bear?"* (Proverbs 18:14). I was walking out in faith the things I knew to be true in God's Word about my health. The third thing this doctor said was just as powerful: "You're surrounded by a loving wife, family, and people who love you." I like that prescription. I am blessed that a doctor recognized God's work in my health enough to say, "This is what I can say about you, and it has nothing to do with my medical expertise."

Years ago, I read an interesting article by Dean Ornish, MD, that supports what my doctor recognized about *the healing element of love*: "Love and intimacy are at the root of what makes us sick and what makes us well.... Study after study find that people who feel lonely are many times more likely to get cardiovascular disease than those who have a strong sense of connection and community."[12] Later, in the same article, he goes on to say, "I'm not aware of any other factor in medicine—not diet, not smoking, not exercise, not stress, not genetics, not drugs, not surgery—that has a greater impact on our quality of life, incidence of illness and premature death."[13] To Dr. Ornish and a growing number of other scientists, the real epidemic

---

12. Dean Ornish, MD, "Love Is Real Medicine," *Newsweek*, October 2, 2005, https://www.newsweek.com/love-real-medicine-121033.
13. Ibid.

in American culture is not heart disease but rather emotional and spiritual diseases associated with the heart: alienation, depression, and loneliness.

We have said the same things for years because the Bible says so: *"There is no fear in love; but perfect love casteth out fear: because fear hath torment. He that feareth is not made perfect in love"* (1 John 4:18).

BE AN OVERCOMER

You can see that I have gone through my own valley of the shadow of death. I was shocked at first that I had a heart attack, but I shouldn't have been. It opened my eyes to the truth that I wasn't free from all of the iniquity I had in my own life. I had some stuff that I had buried because I believed I could be an overcomer in spite of it. I was wrong. None of us is an overcomer *in spite of it*—we're overcomers because we deal with it. Then, it doesn't have a right to rule over us. Satan's lies may tempt us, but we just don't listen anymore.

In the years after the heart attack, I have learned the importance of maintaining a proper perspective on life. Our focus cannot be on avoiding death. We have to embrace life daily. The members of the medical community are expert at monitoring and diagnosing issues related to our bodies, but they cannot address our spirituality. They can tell us how to improve our lives through bodily maintenance, but they cannot instruct us on *why* we are alive nor God's purposes for us.

Through my years of study to help people, I have developed insights into cardiovascular disease. However, what was fascinating in my case was a genetic component. I did not have any other peripheral diseases, but I had a genetic susceptibility to fissuring of my arteries. Fissuring are essentially cracks, and this roughening of the inside of the arteries makes it easier for plaque to stick to it. This fissuring led to a buildup of plaque over time, causing the heart attack. It was the reason why I had to have heart surgery in Trinidad and Tobago.

When I looked at cardiovascular disease and my family history, I did not realize there could be this sort of genetic component. Every man in my family tree has died of heart disease. My father and grandfather both died of heart attacks. My father had three heart attacks, and the last one killed him. I should have recognized that something could trigger that part of my family history. Prior to the heart attack there were no clear signs of danger, but this generational vulnerability remained in my life.

WHAT YOU HAVE BEEN PROMISED

Are you buying into the death culture taking hold of the world? People are giving up on their health by making statements such as, "I'm just getting old." Don't let those words dwell in your heart or come out of your mouth! You've bought into a mindset. I've seen so many people buy into a spirit of death. A spirit of death feeds humans with thoughts of death and dying. Some people resign themselves to death or believe there is no reason to keep living. Many people directly equate aging with death. Certainly, we will all die one day as we age, but to only equate aging with death is to omit the importance of living every day unto the Lord!

I want to remind you of what you've been promised. Psalm 90, written by Moses but inspired by God, is your promise: *"The days of our years are threescore years and ten; and if by reason of strength they be fourscore years, yet is their strength labour and sorrow; for it is soon cut off, and we fly away"* (Psalm 90:10).

God tells us that the longevity of man shall be *"threescore years and ten."* That's seventy years. Then, *"if by reason of strength...fourscore."* That's eighty years. Moses goes on in verse 12, *"So teach us to number our days, that we may apply our hearts unto wisdom."* You need to plan on living out your time—and to do it in wisdom!

My point is, aging is not an excuse to check out on life. Moses was eighty before he even started his ministry. He was eighty when the Lord called him to lead Israel out of captivity and pastor a church of two and a half million people! In the kingdom of God, there is no such thing as retirement. You serve others, and you serve Father God, until you fly away!

THE NEED FOR A FATHER'S LOVE

It's amazing how complacent we sometimes become in our self-righteousness, not knowing there are things we need to pay attention to. I didn't have a heart attack because of high cholesterol. Instead, I inherited something in my generation that the men in my family have struggled with, which is an identity problem. The men in my family never gave or received love—even my father, who was a pastor. I never once heard him say to me, "I love you." In fact, as an only child, I was abused by my father physically, verbally, and emotionally.

The men in my family have all been overwhelmed by self-hatred, rage, and anger. My father was a "rage-aholic." I suffered a great deal of physical abuse from him. One time, just because I was listening to a recording of Beethoven in my bedroom, I received such a severe beating that I had to be taken to the doctor for my bones to be reset. I left home as a senior in high school to protect my sanity and my life.

Because of my father's rage and anger, you couldn't get me in a church, for any reason, for twenty years. It was a long, dry place. I was thirty-eight years old before God's love finally penetrated my wounded shell, and I became a believer in Jesus Christ. So, I know victimization. But I also know freedom in the name and person of Jesus Christ. I'm not bitter, because I met my heavenly Father, who is different and who loves me. I did, however, struggle with self-esteem, even with my success over the years. There was still a war going on inside of me that was a disease-maker. I thought what I was practicing was enough, but I got nailed.

I inherited cardiomyopathy from family members who lived before me. Because of a hardening of the blood vessels, the interior lining of my arteries near my heart developed fissures and cracks. The plaque that flowed through my blood vessels caught behind those fissures and began to clog my arteries. So, even though it was not high blood pressure or cholesterol that caused my blocked arteries, the results were the same.

Praise God, what the devil meant for destruction, God turned to good. After I had the heart attack, I became more thoughtful, more understanding, more open to working out my own salvation with fear and trembling. As the Father reforms my heart, I will teach others the truth of how we can be released from the spiritual roots of disease that are after our destruction. I named this my "Journey of Reformation." I need a T-shirt that says, "Remodeling in progress. Excuse my dust!"

Let me encourage you. If your earthly father treated you poorly or neglected you, do not continue to harbor a grudge toward him. It is time to repent to Father God for bitterness and anger toward that father and forgive him. Humans generally only give out what they have received. If someone abused you, it is most likely because they have received the same abuse in their lifetime. The only way we may end this cycle is by repenting of bitterness toward an earthly father and making the choice to trust that Father God loves us by faith in His Word.

THE NUMBER ONE KILLER

Let's look more closely at cardiovascular disease, which has reached epidemic proportions in the United States. Heart disease is still the number one killer in America. According to the American Heart Association, in recent years, cardiovascular disease has accounted for nearly 840,000 deaths each year in the U.S. That's about one out of every three deaths in the country. Roughly 2,300 Americans die of cardiovascular disease each day, which is an average of one death every thirty-eight seconds! Approximately every forty seconds, another American will have a heart attack![14]

Why is this happening? The Bible speaks often about the significance of the heart. One of the most important verses on the heart is Proverbs 4:23, where God warns us that we must *"keep,"* or guard, our hearts *"with all diligence"*: *"Keep thy heart with all diligence; for out of it are the issues of life."*

What flows from our heart? Physically, our heart is the organ that pumps the blood of life through our bodies. Spiritually, the heart is the central residence of our spirit. We need to learn to guard our heart and protect the very issue (source) of our life.

My son, attend to my words; incline thine ear unto my sayings. Let them not depart from thine eyes; keep them in the midst of thine heart. For they are life unto those that find them, and health to all their flesh. Keep thy heart with all diligence; for out of it are the issues of life.

(Proverbs 4:20–23)

14. "Heart Disease and Stroke Statistics 2018 At-a-Glance," https://healthmetrics.heart.org/wp- content/uploads/2018/02/At-A-Glance-Heart-Disease-and-Stroke-Statistics-2018.pdf.

We have the blessing of health when we are walking in obedience to God's Word. When you bring God into the equation of heart health, everything changes for the better. If you are suffering from heart disease or are a likely candidate for it in the future, Father God wants to change your course direction, and He has granted me the privilege of showing you how.

THE MAJOR ROOTS OF HEART DISEASE

The major, underlying spiritual roots of heart disease are anger, rage, fear (producing anxiety and stress), and hardness of heart.

In my decades of reviewing case studies through For My Life retreats, I have observed that people who embrace anger and rage as a lifestyle are very susceptible to heart disease. Anger lies "boiling" just below the surface of their personalities and is triggered by both major and minor incidents. Tempers explode, with outbursts of screaming, throwing objects, and striking out physically at others. Since anger and rage begin with tempting thoughts and feelings from Satan's kingdom enticing us to embrace the law of sin, they will affect our minds *and* bodies, creating dis-ease of function.

I have seen how rage and anger lead to high cholesterol. Anger affects nervous system activity and raises blood pressure. The risk of a heart attack doubles for two hours after an episode of intense anger. Ongoing hostility, just like ongoing fear, brings with it an avalanche of stress hormones that compromise the immune system.

At Be in Health, we have also found that Type A personalities have a greater tendency toward anger. Since the mid-1970s, cardiologists have recognized the Type A personality as being more aggressive, ambitious, controlling, competitive, and impatient than other people, and therefore more prone to heart disease.[15] Some people may believe these personality characteristics are positive, but aggressiveness, a controlling nature, and impatience are not listed as fruits of the Holy Spirit. I was influenced by my own father to have a Type A personality. As a result, I have had to make changes in my own spiritual makeup and personality and shed a lot of things in my life that were not good for me. If you believe these personality traits are positive and not sinful, I suggest reconsidering your position

---

15. Saul McLeod, "Type A and B Personality," Simple Psychology, https://www. simplypsychology.org/personality-a.html.

by comparing them to the list in Galatians, chapter 5: *But the fruit of the Spirit is love, joy, peace, longsuffering, gentleness, goodness, faith, meekness, temperance: against such there is no law"* (Galatians 5:22–23).

Some people actually become addicted to strong emotions like fear, anger, and rage. It becomes a part of them and their personality. My father was addicted to rage. He fed off the adrenaline rush that came with exploding, and it was an integral part of the way he behaved on a regular basis. If that is you, you need to look to God's Word and His ways to break away from the law of sin that has led to these addictive thoughts. Your addiction is whatever you set your affections on other than God.

In many families, lashing out in anger and rage is a protection mechanism. People may feel vulnerable and afraid if they do not explode in anger, but in that moment, it is faith toward God that will sustain them. If someone shames or demeans you for not engaging in a fight or defending yourself, the Bible tells you not to repay evil for evil, despite how you may feel. The apostle Paul instructs us, *"Recompense no man evil for evil. Provide things honest in the sight of all men"* (Romans 12:17). Two verses later, he says, *"Dearly beloved, avenge not yourselves, but rather give place unto wrath: for it is written, Vengeance is mine; I will repay, saith the Lord"* (Romans 12:19).

OVERCOMING ANGER AND RAGE

It is vital to overcome anger and rage. According to 1 John, chapter 3, anger is a serious spiritual defect with serious consequences: *"Hereby perceive we the love of God, because he laid down his life for us: and we ought to lay down our lives for the brethren"* (1 John 3:16).

Remember, forgiving others first begins with understanding the love Father God has extended to us. To keep from becoming frustrated in situations or from lashing out in anger and rage toward others, we must embrace the forgiveness that has been extended toward us. For those of you who struggle with believing Father God has forgiven you, you may need to repent to Him of following after self-hatred, which reminds you of past failures and beats you up for them. You may also need to repent of a spirit of guilt telling you that you cannot be forgiven and a spirit of shame causing you to feel unworthy of God. We have to know and accept this truth of

God's Word in order to be set free. This is the cause and effect of the gospel of Jesus Christ.

DO NOT HARDEN YOUR HEART

There are several verses in the Bible that show us the importance of not hardening our hearts. Because of the spirit-soul-body connection, I believe that the Lord is concerned with both the spiritual and the physical hardening of our hearts. Psalm 95:8 says, *"Harden not your heart, as in the provocation, and as in the day of temptation in the wilderness."*

The question is, what does it mean to harden your heart? The following verses from Psalm 95 give us a clue: *"When your fathers tempted me, proved me, and saw my work. Forty years long was I grieved with this generation, and said, It is a people that do err in their heart, and they have not known my ways: unto whom I sware in my wrath that they should not enter into my rest"* (Psalm 95:9–11).

When a person doubts and argues with God and His Word, they are not at peace and rest. If you will not trust God and obey His Word, if you continually doubt it, you only have one recourse—to become your own "god." Paul identified that this kind of doubt and unbelief was behind the hardheartedness of Israel in the wilderness. And Hebrews 3:12 says, *"Take heed, brethren, lest there be in any of you an evil heart of unbelief, in departing from the living God."*

Another component behind a hard heart is a spirit of rebellion. A person with a spirit of rebellion is not teachable. They will not listen to correction and will not bend to the Word of God. Having a hard heart is reflective of being rebellious against God and rejecting His Word. Without God's instruction, we have no hope. We are left to follow the world's opinions or figure out how to deal with life's circumstances on our own, which will not satisfy us or bring the help and provision we truly need. *"For rebellion is as the sin of witchcraft, and stubbornness is as iniquity and idolatry. Because thou hast rejected the word of the* LORD, *he hath also rejected thee from being king"* (1 Samuel 15:23).

You will not find peace or rest if you try to take care of yourself and all your own needs. But when you choose to heed Father God's instruction without arguing about it and doubting it, you release yourself to His loving and all-sufficient care. Allow the love and peace of God to rule and reign in your heart. He is your answer to a hardened heart. With heart problems, people have lost their peace and lost their way; they have very troubled hearts. Jesus is offering us His peace, a peace that is beyond any other the world can offer. He says, *"Peace I leave with you, my peace I give unto you: not as the world giveth, give I unto you. Let not your heart be troubled, neither let it be afraid"* (John 14:27).

To have that kind of peace, we need to trust the Lord and rest in Him. Believe and embrace His love for you. Heed Hebrews 3:15: *"While it is said, To day if ye will hear his voice, harden not your hearts, as in the provocation."* I am thankful and grateful for everything in my life today. I truly appreciate and love my wife, and I appreciate the extension of life that God has given me to spend with her on this earth. She is my dearest friend in life.

I want to keep my heart soft and open to the Lord and to His voice. I don't ever want to hear the words "Henry, I never knew you," as Jesus spoke about in Matthew 7:23: *"And then will I profess unto them, I never knew you: depart from me, ye that work iniquity."*

We need to be teachable for God. He is our Father. We are His offspring—sons and daughters. That means relationship. He is our *"Abba, Father"*: *"For ye have not received the spirit of bondage again to fear; but ye have received the Spirit of adoption, whereby we cry, Abba, Father"* (Romans 8:15).

The church is supposed to be an organism, not an organization. God wants every member of the body of Christ to be in relationship with Him and with one another. He is after that relationship with us as our Father, just like He was all the way back to Adam and Eve in the cool of the garden.

A SPIRIT OF FEAR AND OUR HEART

The Bible says that in the last days, men's hearts will fail them because of fear: *"Men's hearts failing them for fear, and for looking after those things which are coming on the earth: for the powers of heaven shall be shaken"* (Luke 21:16).

Most interpretations of this verse only focus on the future catastrophic events to come. However, there are enough fearful events taking place in the world today for us to apply this Scripture to our own lives. The hearts of men and women are failing them because of fear. We are afraid of the future, afraid of one another, afraid of political outcomes, and afraid of illness. We are plagued by the fear of death. We may not be aware of a spirit of fear in our lives, but are we stressed and anxious on an ongoing basis? Remember, that is the physiological evidence of a spirit of fear. It is important to remember that stress is the opposite of peace. Living in peace is a wonderful by-product of trusting God with our life and our future.

Through the ministry, we have observed that the first target organ for the spiritual roots of fear is the heart. Remember, the enemy cannot give you a cardiovascular disease just by tempting you with thoughts of fear unless you give him permission. Jesus finished the work for us on the cross. If only we could apply, in its entirety, what He accomplished for us, we could overcome all such temptation. Unfortunately, we are not perfect, and we are on a journey of applying truth day by day. Now, we need to make daily decisions to follow the Word of God in obedience. This means that even when you are tempted to focus on and become fearful of a bad circumstance, you must make the decision to choose Father God instead. You may have to make this decision moment by moment and day by day, but as you learn to set your heart to trust Father God, it will become a more natural part of your life.

This is what it looks like to live in faith and *not* in fear. You are the one responsible for the cause and effect. You are responsible to respond to God and His Word; you are not responsible to respond to the devil. Hebrews 5:14 says, *"Even those who by reason of use have their senses exercised to discern both good and evil."*

Christians must learn to discern both good and evil. You cannot say, "The devil made me do it." You have the responsibility to seek God's Word in order to make the right decision. That is cause and effect. The Bible tells us, *"For in him we live, and move, and have our being; as certain also of your own poets have said, For we are also his offspring"* (Acts 17:28).

We live in this world, but we don't have to act like the world. Take on God's nature instead. Repent of, and put off, Satan's nature, which is creating disease in your body.

SPECIFIC HEART DISEASES

Let's look at some specific cardiovascular diseases and the spiritual roots behind them.

HYPERTENSION

Spiritual:

Spirits of fear of tomorrow and projecting fear into the future. Our primary reference is found in Matthew 6:34, which reads, *"Take therefore no thought for the morrow: for the morrow shall take thought for the things of itself. Sufficient unto the day is the evil thereof."*

Soul/Thoughts:

People who are entertaining thoughts from this spirit of fear (fear of tomorrow/projecting fear into the future) may manifest worry in every area of their life: family, health, politics, vocation, etc. It is the lack of trust and peace in God's provision and direction that leads to the consistent worrying about such things.

Body/Physical:

Hypertension is the medical term for high blood pressure. Hypertension is sustained elevation of resting systolic blood pressure, diastolic blood pressure, or both. Now, I know that some cases of hypertension are a side effect of certain other diseases, like type 1 diabetes, but these roots pertain to primary hypertension.

Specific Insights:

According to the American Heart Association, "an estimated 103 million U.S. adults have high blood pressure…. That's nearly half of all adults in the United States."[16] This is a plague that we can stop if we will embrace God's truth concerning how to overcome fear and anxiety in our lives. That's why it is so important to understand how the spirit-soul-body connection and temptation affect your biology. Cast down those temptations and unwanted thoughts of fear and stress from the enemy, repent to

16. "More Than 100 Million Americans Have High Blood Pressure, AHA says," American Heart Association News, https://www.heart.org/en/news/2018/05/01/ more-than-100-million-americans- have-high-blood-pressure-aha-says.

the Lord of embracing that law of sin, renew your mind with the truths of God's Word, and meditate on the Scriptures that tell us not to fear or be anxious about anything.

To treat high blood pressure, doctors prescribe pills that are called beta blockers. They cause the blood vessels to relax, which allows the blood to return to its natural flow. Taking medicine will bring your body back into balance and control high blood pressure, but it won't heal you of the underlying cause. God's will is for you to get rid of the fear, anxiety, and stress for good. Now, I'm not telling you to stop taking your blood pressure medicine. But as you embrace the truth of God's Word and experience freedom from fear, your doctor may eliminate that medicine from your life.

ANGINA PECTORIS
Spiritual:

Angina pectoris stems from a spirit of fear, as referenced in the gospel of Luke, which causes a human's heart to fail. *"Men's hearts failing them for fear, and for looking after those things which are coming on the earth: for the powers of heaven shall be shaken"* (Luke 21:26).

Soul/Thoughts:

The spirit of fear leads the person to "feel" like they have to perform to make everything right, especially around their workplace, for example.

Body/Physical:

Angina pectoris is chest pain that occurs because the heart is not receiving enough blood and oxygen, usually due to the thickening of the arteries near the heart. Patients feel heaviness, pressure, or very painful spasms in the chest as a result of stress or physical exertion.

HEART ARRHYTHMIAS
Spiritual:

This condition stems from a spirit of rejection with the manifestation of fear of man, fear of rejection, and rebellion.

Soul/Thoughts:

A person who does not "feel" accepted can begin to strive to be accepted, wanted, and loved. If someone does not respond to them in the affirmative, fear of rejection manifests as wondering "What did I do wrong?" Fear of man says, "I'd better do it the way they want me to." Rebellion (hardness of heart) is the final outcome when there appears to be no way to be accepted. It may say, "Because there is no way to be accepted, I will not listen to anyone and will do what I choose instead."

Body/Physical:

Heart arrhythmias are due to an electrical breakdown in the heart rate. They are disturbances of the heart rhythm, with the spiritual roots of fear, anxiety, and stress. Because of the spirit-soul-body connection, and the disturbances that wrong thoughts can cause to bodily systems, the cardiovascular system does not receive the correct electrical signals, and the heartbeat is interrupted.

MITRAL VALVE PROLAPSE

Spiritual:

This condition is caused by a spirit of shame with the armor of rejection, including insecurities, fear of failure, fear of the future, and dread.

Soul/Thoughts:

People with mitral valve prolapse feel unworthy and diminished in who they are because of shame. As a result, they feel like nobody wants them and that they are unacceptable (a spirit of rejection). As a result of these feelings of shame and unworthiness (rejection), such people are likely to experience fear (stress and anxiety) and insecurities.

Body/Physical:

With heart disease, we have discovered that in many cases, the mitral valve stays open or closed because of neurological misfirings that are similar to arrhythmias. These misfirings interrupt the electrical connection to the valve.

ANEURYSMS

Spiritual:

Whenever I find a person with exploding or bulging blood vessels, I find spirits of anger and rage.

Soul/Thoughts:

A person with spirits of anger and rage will explode when triggered by certain life events. Anger and rage are evidence of bitterness in a person's life. Therefore, there is a tendency to hold a record of wrongs (unforgiveness), which means they will dwell on thoughts of past offenses committed against them. This will stir up intense feelings of anger and rage and the desire to repay evil for evil.

Body/Physical:

An aneurysm is an abnormal, balloon-like swelling in the side of an artery caused by a weakness in the arterial wall. It can be in the brain or in the heart; either way, it involves either the swelling or the rupturing of blood vessels. Varicose veins are another form of an aneurysm.

CORONARY ARTERY DISEASE (ATHEROSCLEROSIS)

Spiritual:

This disease stems from a spirit of self-hatred coming from a lack of proper love, leading to a spirit of fear causing insecurities and pride (which is false confidence).

Soul/Thoughts:

Thoughts like "I can't do anything right" and "I can never measure up" come from a spirit of self-hatred. More than anything else, it is a love issue from a lack of love and nurturing. When a person is not told "I love you" by anyone and is not hugged appropriately (starting in childhood), they develop a stiffening/insecurity about their value.

Body/Physical:

This is the number one cause of heart attacks. Primarily, it involves a blockage of the arteries near the heart so that oxygen is prevented from reaching the heart muscle. Coronary artery disease also involves the hardening of the arteries, which leads to a narrowing of those arteries and restriction of blood flow. For years, all narrowing of the arteries was blamed on cholesterol buildup of plaque. However, I have seen from my own heart attack, and from the case histories of others, that there are spiritual roots that are also the culprit of plaque buildup.

CARDIOMYOPATHY

Spiritual:

Cardiomyopathy is a result of having a spiritually hard heart, such as is consumed with the spirits of doubt, unbelief, and rebellion. Hard-hearted people need to keep their hearts open to God's reproof.

Soul/Thoughts:

This person may struggle with being corrected or told when they are wrong, either by other humans or as they read the Bible. They may also have thoughts that question the Word of God and doubt whether it is true or relevant to them.

Body/Physical:

Cardiomyopathy is a disease of the heart muscle. In most cases, cardiomyopathy causes the heart muscle to become enlarged, thick, or rigid. The heart doesn't function normally and struggles to beat. The blood vessels can become hardened, as well, and develop cracks and fissures.

CEASE FROM ANGER

The Word of God has a great deal to say about anger and rage. The Psalms tell us that the Lord is slow to anger and abounding in lovingkindness. This is your road map to learning to partake of God's nature. Psalm 103:8 says, "*The LORD is merciful and gracious, slow to anger, and plenteous in mercy.*" If we desire to be children of Father God, we must come to terms with the need to repent of anger and bitterness because those attributes are not a part of His character.

None of us wants to be considered a fool. Whenever someone is stirred up in anger, they do not appear to be wise. They look foolish. Not only that, but, in many cases, they will regret what they said and did when bitterness took hold of them and they lashed out toward others. Bitterness and anger bring shame because they do not exalt a person who appears unhinged. We cannot afford to be controlled by anger. It will destroy our bodies in the end. The Word warns us, "*Be not hasty in thy spirit to be angry: for anger resteth in the bosom of fools*" (Ecclesiastes 7:9).

What should we do instead? We should learn to forgive others despite the offenses they commit against us. The more we practice releasing to Father God any transgressions done against us, the less power Satan's kingdom has to tempt us. It will be your glory to pass over a transgression and forgive the one who has sinned against you, just as Jesus has us do when we pray the Lord's Prayer.

Proverbs 19:11 says, "*The discretion of a man deferreth his anger; and it is his glory to pass over a transgression.*" When we allow ourselves to manifest rage and anger, the Bible says we are "*like a city that is broken down, and without walls*": "*He that hath no rule over his own spirit is like a city that is broken down, and without walls*" (Proverbs 25:28).

Learn to rule over your own spirit, in Jesus's name. When you feel angry and have thoughts of offenses done against you, it is time to pause and consider where these thoughts are coming from. Who is speaking to you? Is a spirit of bitterness trying to ensnare you? Do not allow your city to be broken down; do not give the enemy easy access to you because your walls of faith have broken down.

I want you to win this battle in your life. Will you pray with me right now?

Father, thank You for Your Word, which takes us beyond science to the full truth. Thank You for warning us that anger, rage, hostility, stress, fear, anxiety, and hard-heartedness can have a direct impact on our cardiovascular health. God, You are greater than our sin. First John 3:20 says, "*For if our heart condemn us, God is greater than our heart, and knoweth all things.*" Therefore, Lord, even if our heart condemns us, You are greater than our sin. And if we confess our sins and repent of them, Your Holy Spirit will help us with a reformation in our personalities. In Jesus's name, amen.

HEALED OF HYPERTENSION AND INTERSTITIAL CYSTITIS

DOUG AND CARRIE

If you had told us a year ago about all of the changes that would occur in our lives over the next twelve months, we never would have believed you. There were so many areas of our lives that just felt "stuck," and we had accepted them as "just the way things are."

Doug had hypertension, and his blood pressure was spiking to dangerous levels. He often felt hopeless and depressed about the future. My chronic urinary tract infections had led to interstitial cystitis (an ongoing inflammatory condition in the bladder), and I was often in immense pain for days at a time. The only relief I had was from special medicine that had to be administered through a catheter. Both of us had incredible amounts of fear, anxiety, stress, and anger about all of the situations we found ourselves in. It was affecting our marriage and spilling over to our children.

We had the book *A More Excellent Way* sitting on our bookshelf for thirteen years but never had any desire to look at it. Finally, when we had already tried every other modality for healing, we figured it couldn't hurt. When we finished reading, we knew we had to attend a For My Life retreat together.

Even though we had been in Christian ministry for years, now, for the first time, we truly believed in the Father's love for us. We recognized many of the strongholds that were affecting us and our children, and we learned how to change through meaningful repentance combined with resisting Satan's law of sin.

A lot happened in that first week, and we came home overflowing with hope. Back at home, we kept at it by putting the principles we had learned into practice. A couple of months later, I went back to Be in Health for the Walk Out Workshop and received great insight into how to overcome the strongholds of fear, rejection, and bitterness. We went back again for the family week, so that all four of our children could attend the kids' program and hear about the Father's love for themselves.

Learning the truth about healing and disease through the Be in Health ministries completely changed our lives. Although we are just in the beginning of our journey, we are so grateful to have found these biblical truths in this season of our lives. Doug's blood pressure is much lower, he has been healed of food allergies, and he is more engaged in the godly order of our home. I am off all of my medication, and my bladder pain has subsided substantially. We know this journey of overcoming isn't always easy, but we are committed to knowing the Father's love and desire for us. And our lives are improving more and more each day.

NINE

THE SPIRITUAL ROOTS OF MENTAL ILLNESS

The world is filled with despair and anger. Many people feel as though they have no hope. If we have been born again, we should have joy because of our relationship with the Godhead. After all, as believers, we have the joy of the Lord as our strength!

Then he said unto them, Go your way, eat the fat, and drink the sweet, and send portions unto them for whom nothing is prepared: for this day is holy unto our LORD: neither be ye sorry; for the joy of the LORD is your strength. (Nehemiah 8:10)

We are sons and daughters of the living God, and we are joint-heirs with Jesus Christ. We have hope beyond this lifetime extending into the eternal future. Then why do some Christians struggle with hopelessness, depression, and despair? The Bible tells us that the joy of the Lord is our strength. But, too often, God's people are unhappy wanderers. We should be the joy of the planet and the salt and the light of the world. Why aren't we?

Your spirituality directly affects every part of your physical body, and that includes your brain. I don't want to get too involved in the clinical aspects of mental illness, but I do want to uncover the spiritual roots of disease that can affect the mind.

Throughout this book, you have learned that you are a triune being—you are a spirit, you have a soul, and you live in a body. This is a foundational truth for the healing of all disease, including mental illness. Diseases of the mind begin the same way as other diseases. The enemy begins to infiltrate your thoughts with temptations and lies from within. When you embrace those lies as truth instead of believing the Word of God, your mind will be affected. Anytime you do not deal with thoughts from the enemy that are a part of the law of sin, those thoughts will eventually become part of your personality. Remember that Satan's kingdom knows how to train you in mood disorders. The enemy knows how to entrap you through temptation.

WHAT IS DEPRESSION?

Depression is defined as a mental health disorder that involves your thoughts, your behavior, your feelings, and your sense of well-being. People who are depressed feel consistently sad, anxious, and empty. They may also feel hopeless, helpless, worthless, guilty, irritable, ashamed, or restless. They often lose interest in activities that were once pleasurable to them and may overeat or experience a loss of appetite. They may have problems sleeping, concentrating, and making decisions. Withdrawal and isolation are some of the worst results of depression.[17]

Biologically, depression is defined as a chemical imbalance in the body. There is nothing organically wrong with the brain, but there is a disruption in the normal function of the brain's neurotransmitters, so that they fail to secrete the correct balance of three brain chemicals: *serotonin, dopamine*, and *norepinephrine*. The homeostasis, or balance, of these brain chemicals is affected. Over a period of time, mental illness and disorders are the result.

Science does not recognize just one cause of depression; instead, it says that depression is a result of a combination of factors. One factor may be heredity; a part of your family tree can make you more susceptible to the

---

17. American Psychiatric Association, *Diagnostic and Statistical Manual of Mental Disorders*, 5th ed. (Arlington, VA: American Psychiatric Publishing, 2013), 160–161.

triggers that interfere with the brain's chemical balance. Other factors are environmental issues, psychological elements, or the side effects of certain medications. However, one thing science does not acknowledge is the influence of evil spirits, which are often the root cause of mental illness.

THE SPIRITUAL ROOTS OF DEPRESSION

Science focuses on the brain, otherwise known as the psyche or soul. When addressing depression, scientists focus on counseling the soul. However, what many For My Life attendees dealing with depression have discovered at our retreat is the need to get rid of the evil spirit influencing their thoughts. We have heard countless testimonies of those freed from depression when they repented of having followed after the thoughts of evil spirits. You must decide not to listen to those thoughts any longer. In order to become free from torment, you need to repent of following evil spirits, have them cast out, and then cast down the evil thoughts in the future. You must bring them captive to the obedience of Jesus Christ, *"casting down imaginations, and every high thing that exalteth itself against the knowledge of God, and bringing into captivity every thought to the obedience of Christ"* (2 Corinthians 10:5).

I have found several spiritual roots behind depression. The spirits of self-accusation, self-introspection, and self-centeredness are the enemies of someone struggling with depression. The spirit of self-accusation accuses the individual of being the origin of the sin that is tearing their life down. The person fails to recognize that evil spirits are at the root. Self-introspection and self-centeredness focus a person's attention on themselves and their negative thoughts, inhibiting their ability to place their faith and attention on Father God.

These spirits are coupled with shame and guilt. Shame makes a person feel devalued, and guilt will not allow them to believe that they can be forgiven for their sin. Self-pity is the glue that holds it all together. If you struggle with self-pity, then you are struggling with faith. I like to call self-pity the "superglue of hell" binding you to your past (failures). It frequently reflects the failure of something in the past that you are constantly reliving by bringing it into the present.

Serotonin is also depleted in individuals who do not feel loved and accepted. In such situations, because of the spirit-soul-body connection, the hypothalamus and other parts of the limbic system are then affected—those glands responsible for regulating mood, thinking, sleep, appetite, and behavior. Important chemicals the brain needs to function correctly are thrown out of balance. All the enemy needs to do is manipulate your biochemistry to create this havoc. Once again, he does it through the influence of thought. His kingdom of darkness gives you a thought, convinces you that this thought comes from you, and then pressures you to agree with it. In the case of depression, your brain will then conform to those thoughts.

The problem with psychiatry is that it is the practice of medicine apart from an understanding of how God has created us. Practitioners treat their patients as though they only have a soul and a body. They don't acknowledge or understand that we are also a spirit because they can't see the spirit realm. They do not understand that a spiritual influence is the root cause behind many diseases. Remember, it is our observation that spiritual roots are behind approximately 80 percent of diseases and disorders of the mind and body.

DON'T USE MINDLESS MEDITATION

For the treatment of mental disorders, the medical community turns to altered states of consciousness to bring healing, usually in the form of meditation or drugs. Many practitioners will recommend forms of meditation to gain peace over anxiety and stress. Their idea of daily meditation is to let your mind go free. This is New Age teaching. Don't touch it!

Remember, mindless meditation opens the doorway for anything to come into your consciousness. It doesn't teach you anything, but it does leave you wide-open to thoughts and temptations from an evil kingdom. In contrast, the closest form of biblical "meditation" is considering God's Word daily. Do not let your mind go blank in meditation! Meditate on the Word of God. Be like the psalmist, who said, *"I will meditate in thy precepts, and have respect unto thy ways"* (Psalm 119:15).

> *For the word of God is quick, and powerful, and sharper than any two-edged sword, piercing even to the dividing asunder of soul and spirit, and of the joints and marrow, and is a discerner of the thoughts and intents of the heart.*   (Hebrews 4:12)

The Word of God is living and active and is like a two-edged sword that has the power to divide between your soul and your spirit and bring God's truth into your depressed state.

DON'T BE CONDEMNED!

An altered state of consciousness through drug intervention doesn't teach you anything, either. Some patients are prescribed a beta blocker, an antipsychotic drug, or a selective serotonin reuptake inhibitor (SSRI), such as Prozac, which redirects their consciousness so that they are now unaware of the things they don't want to think about. That's why drugs are so powerful—they create these altered states of consciousness.

God doesn't want you to go into an altered state of consciousness. He doesn't even want you to avoid the temptations of your enemy. He wants you to recognize them, face them, and defeat them through the power of His Holy Spirit and His Word. The God of peace is not the god of Prozac. Jesus is the "Prince of Peace."

> *For unto us a child is born, unto us a son is given: and the government shall be upon his shoulder: and his name shall be called Wonderful, Counsellor, The mighty God, The everlasting Father, The Prince of Peace.*   (Isaiah 9:6)

You may live in a world of drugs that block the pathways to depression, but the enemy of your soul is still active in your life. That is not how God wants it to be.

Now, I want to assure you that we are not telling anyone to get off their medication or to feel condemned for being on it! This is not what we teach at all. God is full of grace and mercy. Medications will help manage you and bring you some relief; they are a bridge to your road to freedom. You may need to take an antidepressant temporarily while you apply your heart to the Word of God until you are free of the depression. However, the ultimate goal is for you to no longer need medication one day. The medical profession tries to help keep people going, keep functioning as normally as possible. At Be in Health, we don't want people to just keep going. We want them to be set free!

TAKE OWNERSHIP OF YOUR LIFE

Please do not think I am insensitive to the depths to which depression can take a person or that I am being flippant about the condition. My heart of compassion is to help you to prevent or defeat this condition. Additionally, I am not insinuating that defeating depression is merely mind over matter. When I tell you to "take ownership of your life," that is not mind over matter. That is taking personal responsibility for deciding which kingdom you will serve.

There is a battle over you every day; there is an evil kingdom assigned to interfere with your journey in God. Remember, your battle is not with you or any other person. Your battle is with principalities and powers. It is with invisible beings and spiritual wickedness in high places and the darkness of this world. Your role in the battle is to grab hold of the truth of the Word of God and to be an overcomer. Begin by reading the Scriptures or having someone read them to you. Saturate your mind with the sanity of God's Word. Remember that faith comes by hearing, and hearing by the Word of God: "*So then faith cometh by hearing, and hearing by the word of God*" (Romans 10:17).

Allow the sanity of the Word to overcome the insanity from the enemy that has flooded your mind in the past. It is necessary to renew your mind by God's Word in order to bring chemical balance back into your brain. Biologically, you need to bring the serotonin level up to get the balance back to normal. How does this work? The first step is to recognize that your feelings of hopelessness and despair do not come from yourself or from God—they come from evil spirits belonging to a hidden, destructive kingdom. Acknowledge this fact and repent of accepting these thoughts and feelings that are not based on God's Word. Remember, *"If we confess our sins, he is faithful and just to forgive us our sins, and to cleanse us from all unrighteousness"* (1 John 1:9).

Forgiveness and freedom in Christ will bring peace and joy to your soul and cause your serotonin levels to rise. When you cast down every imagination that raises itself up against the truth of God, your serotonin levels will continue to rise. Your chemistry will begin to regain its balance. Could it really be that simple? Yes, in many cases of depression, I have seen success in this way.

SCIENTIFIC PROOF OF SUCCESS

Be in Health has been blessed with a high success rate in the healing of depression and stress disorders. In 2010, I had a meeting in Kuala Lumpur, Malaysia, with professionals from several countries. We had a lively discussion about the remarkable testimonies of healing of the spirit, soul, and body from our For My Life retreats. They asked me, "Can these impressive results be scientifically measured?"

A year later, Be in Health launched a formal, scientific, three-year physical, mental, and spiritual health study at the For My Life retreats. The study was conducted under the supervision of the human research ethics committee of South Africa's Stellenbosch University, Department of Interdisciplinary Health Sciences, Division of Community Health. The title of the results of the study might seem a little bit intimidating! It is *The Effect of a Faith-Based Education Program (4ML program) on Self-Assessed Physical, Mental and Spiritual (Religious) Health Parameters*—PHYMSH, for short!

Only the attendees of the For My Life retreats who had no previous knowledge of our program were invited to be part of the study. Each of the subjects took four identical surveys at four different times: (1) before the retreat, (2) on the last day of the retreat, (3) one month post-retreat, and (4) four months post-retreat. The areas measured were depression, stress and anxiety, religious coping skills, and illness sensitivity. An important scale measured whether the change would last, indicating a character change for the better. The conclusion by Stellenbosch University was that attendance at the For My Life retreat "produced statistically and clinically significant changes; these lasted in those followed up >1 year."[18]

After the study was completed, Be in Health independently continued to track individuals who had been in the study up to five years post-retreat, and they reported little to no relapse. The results of these interviews produced the following internal statistics:

- 91 percent of major depression was reduced to mild to no depression.

- 90 percent reported a reduction of their stress level.

- 86 percent indicated that stress no longer affected them negatively.

- 88 percent reported a greater ability to cope with illness in general.

- 84 percent reported a more positive outlook on life.

These participants of the For My Life retreat had opened their hearts to God and let Him meet them. God has honored Be in Health with His Word, and thousands have been healed. *"Ye shall know the truth, and the truth shall make you free"* (John 8:32). Accept it. Embrace it.

OTHER INSIGHTS FOR YOUR RECOVERY

Everyone who struggles with depression or any other mental disorder would like the problem to be gone immediately, but you may not come out of depression rapidly just because of this teaching or just because you declare, "I have enough faith to defeat it!" Your mind may have been trained in hopelessness and despair for some time. You will have to walk out your salvation and consistently renew your mind. That is why I am giving you the tools to recover from depression and prevent it from returning.

An important first step to your recovery is to come out of isolation. Depression will take you away from people when you need them the most because they can help you bear your burden. They can read the Word to you or with you. They can pray for you and with you, they can love you, and

---

18. Frans J. Cronjé et al., *Journal of Religion and Health* 56, no. 1 (September 2015), http://www.researchgate.net/publication/282045748_Effect_of_a_Faith-Based_Education_Program_on_Self_Assessed_Physical_Mental_and_Spiritual_(Religious)_Health_Parameters.

they can encourage you, bringing you out of a dark place and showing you that someone really loves you.

Another powerful tool for defeating depression is to read Psalm 139. Now, don't use this psalm as a placebo. Don't read it as though just doing so is a secret formula for healing. You need to believe the Scriptures, to trust in and actively apply them to your life. The power of the Word of God and your decision to embrace it can defeat depression in your life!

HELP FOR BIPOLAR DISORDER

Bipolar disorder, also known as manic-depressive illness, is a brain disorder that causes extreme shifts in mood, energy, activity levels, and the ability to carry out simple tasks. This condition takes the individual through alternating episodes of deep sadness and great elation. Sadness and joy can be a part of the fabric of everyday life, but when they fluctuate in extremes, they are problematic.

Bipolar disorder is often first diagnosed in people between the ages of eighteen and twenty-four as they enter into young adulthood. Heredity seems to be the most important predisposing factor. It is familial, a characteristic of certain families. It especially affects women, who then pass it down genetically to their children. Science has discovered that there may be a defect on the X chromosome that is inherited from the mother. When someone comes to us with a diagnosis of bipolar disorder, I ask them whether their mother or grandmother had it.

The mania part of bipolar disorder is often a fixation on achievement, where people are driven in some uncontrollable way toward success. The mania is actually a form of depression because it involves a drive that can never be satisfied, a black hole that is never filled. Similar to those with depression, people with bipolar disorder always have an imbalance in the chemicals necessary for healthy brain function, particularly a lower level of serotonin.

ROOTS AND RECOVERY OF BIPOLAR DISORDER

To defeat bipolar disorder, you will have to deal with generations of unlovingness. You will have to recognize that this disorder is the product of an unloving spirit, of not feeling accepted, and of being driven to find something to take the place of that lack of acceptance. It is often a result of generations of fathers who did not nurture and love their wives and children. In my years of ministry, I have seen it played out time and time again.

In the bipolar profile, it is the family genes that cause the serotonin in the brain to be greatly diminished. For people who have a predisposition to bipolar disorder, their home and family life must be a safe place of peace to prevent the disorder from manifesting. When a person does not feel safe, loved, or accepted, their body responds by reducing the amount of serotonin, causing additional chemical imbalances.

In the beginning of your recovery from bipolar disorder, the Word of God and the love of God might seem like a small, soft, weak voice. However, as you hear and dwell on God's Word, that voice will become stronger and stronger, and the voice of the enemy will become weaker and weaker, until you make the full exchange and take your life back. In the process, your body will begin to serve you again. The neurotransmitter imbalances will return to normal, and you will no longer have bipolar disorder because the foundation for it will be gone. Freedom with peace of mind is exactly what you will get in exchange.

CAN YOU BE HEALED OF PARANOID SCHIZOPHRENIA?

Paranoid schizophrenia is a compound phobic disorder. It involves paranoia, or fear, and "schizo," which is Latin for "splitting or dividing"—a splitting of the human personality. In paranoid schizophrenia, the person loses touch with reality, often "hearing" voices and having hallucinations. However, in this case, also, there is nothing organically wrong with the brain. The problem lies in the excessive secretion of two neurotransmitters, dopamine and norepinephrine, which causes an extreme fight-or-flight reaction and affects the central nervous system.

As with bipolar disorder, paranoid schizophrenia usually develops in young people who are between eighteen and twenty-four years old. Those who develop the condition generally grew up in families that did not know how to love each other. The fight-or-flight response can begin in a young person who does not feel safe in their family because of abuse or because of extreme pressure to be perfect.

Parents can cause a great deal of damage when they push their children too hard. When one of my children was young, I helped him to avoid a psychiatric disorder when I refused to let him be A-plus oriented just to compete with his friends. I told him, "You're going to be a great student, but you don't have to be an A-plus student. Here's the deal: As, Bs, and Cs are acceptable; Ds and Fs are not. Do the best you can."

Whoever said that all children have to be A-plus students? Because I released my son from that peer and performance pressure, he not only came out of the psychosis that was forming, but he also lost twenty pounds. When he was stuck in the mindset of competition and not liking himself, his rate of metabolism and caloric burn slowed down, making him dislike himself even more. He has gone on to do wonderful things with his life, including excelling in school, but he was saved from a lot of psychological problems that result from performance disorders and fear of failure.

Fear is the spiritual root behind paranoid schizophrenia. It is a tragic example of how fear has torment. Recall 1 John 4:18: "*There is no fear in love; but perfect love casteth out fear: because fear hath torment. He that feareth is not made perfect in love.*"

I consider it not only a phobic disorder, but also a depression disorder, because it involves withdrawal and isolation. If you want to help people who are struggling with their identity and have depressive episodes, including paranoid schizophrenia, start loving them. I know they're hard to get along with, but who asked you to love and get along with only those who are agreeable? Even the heathen can do that!

For if ye love them which love you, what thank have ye? for sinners also love those that love them. And if ye do good to them which do good to you, what thank have ye? for sinners also do even the same....Be ye therefore merciful, as your Father also is merciful.

(Luke 6:32–33, 36)

PERFECT LOVE CASTS OUT FEAR

Years ago, I was teaching about paranoid schizophrenia in the small town of Madison, Minnesota, when a man came up to me and said, "Wow! I have two brothers who were both diagnosed with paranoid schizophrenia. One has already committed suicide. The other brother should be locked up for his own safety. Are you suggesting that if I had loved my older brother, the fear that caused the disorder would have been driven out of him?" I responded, "It's not my suggestion at all. It's what the Word of God says. It says, 'Perfect love casteth out fear.'"

I didn't expect to hear from that gentleman again. Then, a year and a half later, I was teaching a conference in Garland, Texas, when the same man showed up with an incredible testimony. He had driven all the way from Minnesota to Texas just to share his powerful story with me.

He began, "I decided that if the Word of God was true and you were right, rather than avoiding my brother, I would visit him. I'd been avoiding him for a long time because he never made any sense. I couldn't hang out with him because he was out there in his weird world. But I decided I'd give it a shot because I love my brother. Every Saturday, I would give him two or three hours of my time as I tried to find some place of communication with him. I did that every week for an entire year."

This man also shared that, during that year, he never said anything to his brother along the lines of "You need to get it together," or "Stop acting out!" He just showed him his love, with no strings attached. When you tell people who are struggling with mental disorders to "just get it together," they will become worse. You are driving them right into isolation, paranoia, and avoidance. If they could stop their behavior, they would!

The man's story continued, "As I shared my Saturdays with my brother, he became calmer and calmer. Pastor, I need to tell you what happened by the end of that one year. I now have a brother who is in his right mind! He is no longer on any medications. He is engaged to be married, holds a full-time job, and was healed without medical intervention! Pastor, the Word of God is true—perfect love does cast out fear!" This is a testimony to the grace of God and the power of His Word to accomplish what it says it will!

POST-TRAUMATIC STRESS DISORDER

For at least the last fifteen years, there have been many news stories about post-traumatic stress disorder (PTSD). I recently held a conference on PTSD, and thousands of people livestreamed the conference or watched it afterward on our Be in Health website. It was exciting to hear that a number of people received a total healing of their PTSD after the conference just because they now understood the battleground.

PTSD is not a war issue. It is a result of trauma involving fear, anxiety, and stress. People say, "Well, you got PTSD because you went to war," or "Those with PTSD probably grew up in a war zone." But not everybody who is in a war ends up with PTSD.

In our studies, we have found that PTSD involves an enlarged amygdala. Remember that the amygdala is part of the spirit-soul-body connection in the brain. It helps us process feelings and thoughts that come out of the cerebral cortex. The amygdala is the first receiver of highly charged negative thoughts that originate from a spirit of fear. After being hit constantly by these thoughts, the amygdala becomes enlarged or swollen. If the amygdala swells, its ability to rationalize or process functional thought is hindered, and everything comes blasting through, which can cause illness or a psychosis.

When someone who goes to war has a normal amygdala, they can usually process the thoughts, images, and trauma of battle. But for someone who has an enlarged amygdala before they even arrive at the war zone, because of the training of a spirit of fear, their brains will not allow their thoughts to come to a proper conclusion. This condition becomes worse during their time of service.

We have seen people healed of PTSD after they have received God's truth. They needed to come out of isolation and get back into fellowship with people who loved them and could help them. They also had to forgive the person who had hurt them and originally brought on all of the anxiety and fear. First John 4:18 continues to be the word of truth for this situation: *"Perfect love casteth out fear."*

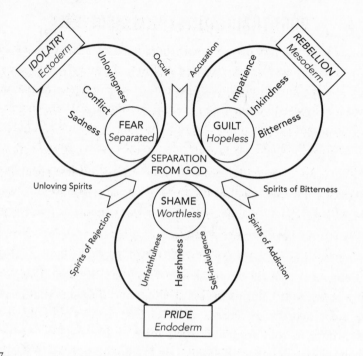

Chart 7

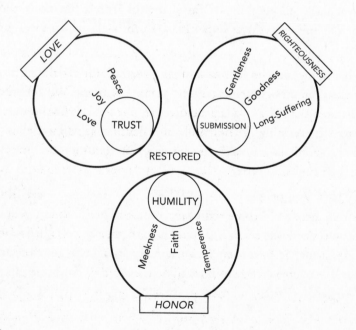

Chart 8

OBSESSIVE-COMPULSIVE DISORDER

Obsessive-compulsive disorder (OCD) is an anxiety and mental health disorder that affects people of all ages and walks of life, but it often begins in childhood and is first detected in early adulthood. OCD always involves a low secretion of serotonin, causing the person to get caught in a cycle of obsessions and compulsions. Obsessions are unwanted, intrusive thoughts, images, or urges that trigger intensely distressing feelings. Compulsions are the behaviors the person uses to quell the unwanted thoughts and feelings.

The spiritual roots behind OCD are guilt and self-hatred. A person who struggles with believing they cannot be forgiven for past failures (guilt)—and has a spirit of self-hatred that beats them up for these same failures—will struggle and feel out of control in their life as if they are sinking. The component of a spirit of fear will tell them that if everything is not in place, something is going to go terribly wrong. To recover, a person with OCD must repent of having a perfectionist mentality, regardless of its origin. They need to believe in, and receive, the heavenly Father's love and forgiveness and begin to trust Him. That is the path to freedom.

THE JOY OF MY SALVATION

We minister to many people who are convinced that there is no hope for their healing from mental disorders. They are filled with self-loathing and depression, and everything those conditions entail. We look them in the eye and say, "Would you repeat after me, please? 'Lord, restore unto me the joy of Your salvation.'" They repeat this statement and then break down in tears because it has often been years since they had any joy. Salvation has not been a joy to them because they have lived under a burden of accusation from the enemy.

Would you do the same right now? Say, out loud, "Lord, restore unto me the joy of Your salvation." Say it again, and then thank and praise God for that truth! *"The kingdom of God is not meat and drink; but righteousness, and peace, and joy in the Holy Ghost"* (Romans 14:17).

Say it out loud: "Joy in the Holy Spirit for me!" Be encouraged by Psalm 126:5–6: *"They that sow in tears shall reap in joy. He that goeth forth and weepeth, bearing precious seed, shall doubtless come again with rejoicing, bringing his sheaves with him."*

Having the mind of Christ is your key to mental health. Your life and mine depend on being willing and able to be changed. God will continue to change us, but we must understand our responsibility. I don't teach anything I haven't had to walk and live. It's not just theory. This is a matter of life and death. You know I have walked in my own valley of the shadow of death. I've learned firsthand the power of God's Word.

Don't be afraid of this battle. God's thinking is superior, and Satan's thinking is inferior. *"Ye are of God, little children, and have overcome them: because greater is he that is in you, than he that is in the world"* (1 John 4:4). Greater is God who is in you than the enemy who is in the world. You choose whom you will serve. God will not leave you or forsake you as you take this journey to freedom!

Be strong and of a good courage, fear not, nor be afraid of them: for the LORD *thy God, he it is that doth go with thee; he will not fail thee, nor forsake thee.*   (Deuteronomy 31:6)

HEALED OF BIPOLAR AND MULTIPLE PERSONALITY DISORDERS

VICKI

I was in and out of psychiatric hospitals for fifteen years. The second time I was admitted to the hospital, a doctor spoke these words over me: "Your life will be a revolving door in and out of psychiatric hospitals." I was first diagnosed with major depression, but then it deteriorated into bipolar disorder, and finally I was diagnosed with multiple personality disorders. I was desperately ill. There was no hope I would ever get better.

Then someone gave me the book *A More Excellent Way*. Soon after, I went to my first For My Life retreat. I had so much to deal with that I attended the retreat a few more times. My husband came with me one of those times because our marriage was a wreck. Both of us had been in torment. Even though he had stood by me through all the years of pain, I knew we had to do this to restore our marriage.

God was so faithful to us! As a result of hearing and applying the biblical teachings on freedom from disease, I have been healed! I am free, absolutely free! No more doctors, no more hospitals, and no more medications at all! Our marriage has been restored. Our God is an awesome God! And the people whom He has used to come into our lives and share these truths with us have been so amazing. I am so very grateful, and I give God all the glory!

TEN

THE SPIRITUAL ROOTS OF
STRESS DISORDERS

There is excessive stress in America. That doesn't surprise you, does it?

The Anxiety and Depression Association of America reports, "Anxiety disorders are the most common mental illness in the U.S., affecting 40 million adults in the United States age 18 and older, or 19.1% of the population every year," with "36.9% of those suffering receiving treatment."[19] A report from the National Institute for Occupational Safety and Health (NIOSH) quotes, "Three-fourths of employees believe that workers have more on-the-job stress than a generation ago."[20]

According to a recent American Psychological Association (APA) survey, the most common sources of stress today are inflation, personal safety, and the future of our nation and the world. As a result, "Around seven in 10 adults (72%) have experienced additional health impacts due to this stress, including feeling overwhelmed, experiencing changes in sleeping habits and/or worrying constantly."[21]

19. "Anxiety Disorders – Facts & Statistics," Anxiety & Depression Association of America, https://adaa.org/about-adaa/press-room/facts-statistics.
20. The National Institute for Occupational Safety and Health (NIOSH), "Stress...At Work," Centers for Disease Control and Prevention, https://www.cdc.gov/niosh/docs/99-101/default.html.
21. "Stress in America 2022: Concerned for the Future, Beset by Inflation," American Psychological Association, October 2022, https://www.apa.org/news/press/releases/stress/2022/concerned-future-inflation.

A CULTURE THAT DEMANDS PERFECTION

In many cultures around the world, people are judged by their performance and accomplishments. From the top levels of government, business, sports, and higher education to domineering, controlling parents in the home, humans are afraid of the shame that comes with failure and mistakes. There is a demand for perfection. There is a pecking order of value, and only the elite performers thrive in education, career, and income, while the rest of us are afraid we will fall by the wayside. This state of affairs creates a lot of stress and anxiety in people's lives. When they internalize this stress, it starts to affect their soul and many of their bodily systems. The result may be that they end up with a stress disorder.

Throughout this section, please keep in mind that today's society may not make provision for failure, but God does! God says that a righteous man will fall and rise again: *"For a just man falleth seven times, and riseth up again: but the wicked shall fall into mischief"* (Proverbs 24:16). Psalm 37:24 encourages us, *"Though he fall, he shall not be utterly cast down: for the LORD upholdeth him with his hand."* And Paul wrote in his second letter to the church at Corinth, *"Therefore I take pleasure in infirmities, in reproaches, in necessities, in persecutions, in distresses for Christ's sake: for when I am weak, then am I strong"* (2 Corinthians 12:10).

WHAT ARE STRESS DISORDERS?

Stress disorders, or syndromes, are a result of a spirit of fear (which manifests as anxiety and stress), along with guilt and shame. With stress disorders, the enemy produces fearful thoughts that cause you to lose your peace. As you dwell on those thoughts, your central nervous system is affected. You begin to experience pain, brain fog, and a host of other symptoms. Medication will simply mask these chemical imbalances, which come are the result of embracing a spirit of fear. Among the most common stress disorders are fibromyalgia, chronic fatigue syndrome, type 2 diabetes, hypertension, irritable bowel syndrome, ulcerative colitis, chronic insomnia, migraines, and acid reflux.

In the face of these fearful thoughts, we must remain aware of the temptation that comes voiced in the first person to convince you to speak against yourself. If only evil spirits came and announced themselves! But, no, they attempt to trick us by giving us thoughts as if those thoughts were our own. A spirit of fear may say, "I am so concerned about what will happen tomorrow."

Remember, Paul wrote, *"For God hath not given us the spirit of fear; but of power, and of love, and of a sound mind"* (2 Timothy 1:7). Unresolved spirits of fear make it impossible to have a sound mind because the mind is hounded by stressful thoughts and imaginations. These individuals cannot give and receive love without fear. We cannot overstate the powerful truth of 1 John 4:18, which states, *"There is no fear in love; but perfect love casteth out fear: because fear hath torment. He that feareth is not made perfect in love."*

If you didn't feel loved during your childhood, you probably won't feel loved by other people as an adult. Guess what joins itself to you when you are not loved correctly? The spirit of fear. I am aware of some people who have a huge breach in their relationships with others because of fear. They are even afraid of the people they go to church with. The person with insecurity and fear walks into a grocery store and becomes afraid when they see the "dreaded" person at the end of the same aisle. They move to the next aisle and peek around the corner to see if the coast is clear! If it is clear, they can breathe again.

The "fear of man" is not the fear of "males" but the fear of people. We are not to be afraid of other humans, but we need to trust Father God because He is our Helper. He is the one we are accountable to for the life we live. When we are afraid of "man," it is a snare or a stumbling block to becoming who God has called us to be. Don't let this be you! Don't be ruled by the fear of man!

The fear of man bringeth a snare: but whoso putteth his trust in the LORD *shall be safe.*   (Proverbs 29:25)

So that we may boldly say, The Lord is my helper, and I will not fear what man shall do unto me.   (Hebrews 13:6)

If you have a fear of others, especially those in your church, you need to repent to Father God. You need to trust Him to build and restore your fellowship with others. If you have avoided people, because of either past conflicts or fear, or because you do not know how to develop relationships, it is time to learn. If there is one place where we must be willing to make mistakes and learn, it is in the church. Jesus taught us to be merciful and forgiving toward one another. If there is one place where we should be learning how to love one another, it is also in the church. As we learn to love, it will drive out the fear because that fear will no longer have an environment to thrive in. It will become a diminishing thought. It will fade into the background because of healthy fellowship with God, yourself, and others. If fear was the underlying root of your stress syndrome, the syndrome will begin to fade away.

SYNDROMES VERSUS DISEASES

Getting rid of spirits of fear is a powerful gateway to freedom from illness. However, we also must understand the physiological problems at the root of stress disorders. At this point, we need to draw a distinction between diseases and syndromes. Both involve an imbalance of homeostasis, but there are physiological differences between them.

At Be in Health, when we use the term *disease*, it is not in a generic way to refer to every malfunction in the body. We define disease as a malfunction where there is *organic damage* to the body—cells have been destroyed and organs have been damaged. On the other hand, with a *syndrome*, we are referring to a dysfunction of a bodily system where *no damage has been done to organs* and *no body parts have been physically destroyed*. In a syndrome, even though there is no apparent disease, a malfunction of undetermined origin is at work—specific parts of the body are not doing their job correctly.

The foundation for healing in stress disorders lies in this understanding of syndromes. Stress disorders are not caused by the destruction of body parts; therefore, they are considered syndromes. I have remarked that syndromes are actually "S-I-N-dromes," since they are brought on by accepting the law of sin into your life. By embracing the lies of Satan for a prolonged period of time, even years, malfunctions appear in your body that are known as syndromes.

Your body is designed to serve you, and it should fulfill that function correctly unless something interferes with its design. When you do not repent of and then cast down temptations from the spirit of fear, you are internalizing fear as the mindset to guide your future decision-making. By this process, the spirit of fear will project potential failure into your future, and you will feel stress and anxiety in your soul and body. Your limbic system responds and your hypothalamus senses that you are not at peace. As a result of entertaining spirits of fear, guilt, or shame, the hypothalamus causes misfired electrical and chemical signals to go out to the rest of the body and cause dis-ease of function in the endocrine system, the nervous system, the digestive system, or all of these systems. One result is multiple stress disorders. At For My Life, we have seen this outcome in thousands of people over years of ministry. You may know someone who suffers from multiple disorders or syndromes, as well.

Medical science has observed that physiological anxiety and stress (which we understand are caused by a spirit of fear) and emotional trauma change the brain, but, for most syndromes, doctors do not know the cause or the cure. That is why they prescribe antidepressants or anti-anxiety medications and supplements, or why they put their patients on holistic alternative protocols. We know the real solution is to align your spirit and soul with the Word of God, to meditate on the Word, and to walk in God's truth until it becomes a part of your long-term memory, replacing the stress-filled lies of the enemy. Then peace—not fear and stress—will reign in your heart and life.

A HEALING OF MULTIPLE STRESS DISORDERS

God still heals today. Even chronic stress disorders that are considered incurable are subject to His Word. At Be in Health, we have seen many people healed of stress disorders when they have applied God's truth concerning health. Emily is a woman who was diagnosed with multiple stress disorders until God healed her. Here is her story:

I was living a very active life until about eleven years ago. I was married with five children, was the owner of my own day spa, and served with my husband in our church. Slowly, I began to experience physical symptoms: unexplained joint pain, fatigue, allergic reactions. I suffered from one illness on top of another. After seeing several specialists, I was diagnosed with fibromyalgia, chronic fatigue disorder, chronic migraines, celiac disease (intolerance to gluten), additional food allergies, and hypoglycemia.

I suffered for nine long years with debilitating illnesses. I tried to function for my family, but I was often bedridden because of the pain. Eventually, I had to sell my business and spend most of my time at home. When I went out, I wore a full face mask to protect myself from the environment. I tried everything I could to get well, but nothing worked—not doctors, medicine, holistic treatments, health diets, special supplements, essential oils, or prayer. Some treatments brought temporary relief, but then I would be right back where I started. It was a nightmare.

Two years ago, I was at my very lowest point. My daughter's wedding was approaching, and I was lying in bed in pain when I turned and looked at my nightstand. There were bottles of supplements and prescription medicines sitting there, but none of them had helped me. I was so sick I could hardly speak. At that moment, I believe I heard God say to me, "Are you ready to do it *My* way?"

A couple of months later, I was at a women's Bible study, telling my story and asking for prayer. Afterward, a woman came up to me and said, "I have something I need to share with you." We talked for two hours, and she shared the biblical truth she learned from Be in Health and the For My Life retreat. She was excited as she explained how God had healed her and set her free through His Word. I knew that God had been preparing me for the words I heard that day.

My husband and I agreed that this was the next step. Two months later, I was in Thomaston, Georgia, at a weeklong For My Life retreat. From the very first day, I heard biblical truth that seemed like it was directed at me. Everything being taught was steeped in the Word of God, and I could clearly see the truth. I was adopted at the age of thirteen, and I realized that there were some things I needed to take care of. The Holy Spirit began working on my heart, bringing back situations, leading me to repent of things in my heart.

My healing was not instantaneous, but by the end of the week, my body was not hurting as much, and I felt as though a great heaviness had lifted off me. I was able to go home with a new understanding of God's Word on healing. I now had a "spiritual toolbox" of discernment that I could use to apply the biblical teachings on healing.

The first week I was home, I decided to eat some of the food I was "allergic" to, in moderation. It was a step of faith for me; I was not going to let fear of those foods keep me down. None of the food bothered me! In the following weeks and months, my health continued to improve without any medical intervention. The pain and fatigue vanished; the allergies disappeared. I am healthier now than I ever was before I got sick!

My husband, who had been so supportive through all those years of sickness, was so thankful, saying, "I have my wife back!" And I can say with joy, "I have my life back! I am so grateful to God!"

Emily is not the only person we have seen at the For My Life retreats who has been diagnosed with multiple stress syndromes. When the immune system is compromised, disorders can attack the body from all sides. Sometimes people will come to us and bring a list of ten or more diseases and syndromes. Of course, they want all ten of them to go away. Let me tell you that there is always one primary disease or syndrome; the rest are peripheral. You will never defeat a secondary illness if you do not defeat the primary illness that spawns the others. When you deal with the primary one, and God heals you, the other nine will disappear automatically.

Folks, these are things you need to hear! We are so busy chasing symptoms and disease profiles that we don't even consider why we got sick to begin with or how we can get better, and our doctors often do not know, either.

STRESS DISORDERS: THEIR ROOTS AND CURES

This section differs slightly from previous sections because not every stress disorder listed has a spirit, soul, and/or body component.

FIBROMYALGIA

Fibromyalgia is a stress and anxiety disorder. Its classic symptoms are pain in the muscles, ligaments, and connective tissue; fatigue; and chronic insomnia. Women make up 99 percent of the people diagnosed with fibromyalgia. Thankfully, we have seen countless women healed from this stress disorder.

Fibromyalgia does not occur randomly. It usually occurs in women who have been victimized. By that, I do not mean that they necessarily have experienced physical abuse, but often a lack of care is just as devastating. Case studies show that it primarily comes from the lack of covering or nurturing by a man, perhaps the father or the husband. These women have a spirit of fear of abandonment that comes into their life because of previous abandonment experiences.

Fibromyalgia afflicts females who do not feel covered, protected, nurtured, or safe, and are always looking over their shoulder. They are driven and anxious, moving the pieces of their lives around to try to find some security and stability that they feel is not coming from their husbands or fathers. In most cases, such women have had the burden of the world on their shoulders. They have been the ones leading the home spiritually, taking care of the children, attending to the finances, and perhaps dealing with recurring crises in the home by themselves. They have been carrying the burden all alone because the men in their lives haven't taken care of any of these needs. As a result, these women have gone down under the stress.

The spiritual root behind fibromyalgia is a spirit of fear producing anxiety, stress, drivenness, and perfectionism. Fibromyalgia is triggered by this spirit of fear in a realm beyond our conscious awareness. When we struggle with the spirit of fear, it disrupts our body systems and initiates nerve impulses through the hypothalamus, which senses there is a problem upstream in the soul and the spirit.

Fibromyalgia does not have a known cause or cure in the medical community. Biblically, we know that the way to eradicate it is to repent of embracing the lies of the enemy and allow God to deliver you from this spirit of fear. The Bible tells us not to be anxious over anything!

Be careful for nothing; but in every thing by prayer and supplication with thanksgiving let your requests be made known unto God. And the peace of God, which passeth all understanding, shall keep your hearts and minds through Christ Jesus. Finally, brethren, whatsoever things are true, whatsoever things are honest, whatsoever things are just, whatsoever things are pure, whatsoever things are lovely, whatsoever things are of good report; if there be any virtue, and if there be any praise, think on these things.   (Philippians 4:6–8)

A truth that is repeated throughout this book is that God has not given us a spirit of fear. In order to be healed of fibromyalgia, repent of embracing the spirit of fear of abandonment that has come into your life. As you cast your cares upon the Lord, you may also need to repent of taking on too many burdens. Learn to trust in God and His love to repair and bring healing to those parts of your life where you have felt alone and abandoned. "[Cast] *all your care upon him; for he careth for you*" (1 Peter 5:7).

In addition, renew your mind with biblical truth so that you never again embrace the law of sin concerning fear of abandonment and anxiety. When peace returns to a woman's soul, the nerve signal from the hypothalamus calms down, and fibromyalgia will be cured. As it says in Isaiah 26:3, "*Thou wilt keep him in perfect peace, whose mind is stayed on thee: because he trusteth in thee.*"

CHRONIC FATIGUE SYNDROME

Chronic fatigue syndrome (CFS) is a stress disorder characterized by extreme fatigue that lasts for months, does not go away with bedrest, and cannot be explained by any underlying medical conditions. Other symptoms of CFS include chronic insomnia, muscle pain, headaches, and reduced concentration and memory. Similar to fibromyalgia, over 95 percent of diagnosed cases of chronic fatigue syndrome are observed in women.

The root is a spirit of fear of rejection, and behind it is a drivenness to earn approval and love from an authority figure, usually a parent. The person seeks to earn this approval and love by being successful in the world. Certain cultures are particularly driven by a need for approval from others through success and performance. To them, failure means a lack of identity and acceptance by others. People from these cultures feel additional pressure to receive approval from their community at large. It becomes a great burden.

According to the medical community, there is no known cause or cure for chronic fatigue syndrome. It is hard to diagnose because the symptoms are so much like those of fibromyalgia or multiple sclerosis. Doctors prescribe ways of relieving the symptoms through medication and stress-reducing activities. As you just read in Emily's testimony, the best prescription is to eliminate the spiritual root cause in your life and become completely healed and free!

The person with chronic fatigue disorder needs to embrace the truth of God's Word. We were fearfully and wonderfully made by God, and that alone is what establishes our value!

I will praise thee; for I am fearfully and wonderfully made: marvellous are thy works; and that my soul knoweth right well.   (Psalm 139:14)

Even if our family will not accept us when we fail, we are not rejected by God when we sin. The cure is to repent, release that drive to succeed for the wrong reasons, and realize you have value. You do not have to earn love. God is love. God will always accept you if you turn to Him. All stress disorders involve leaning on yourself or others to be your source of acceptance instead of trusting God. Do not look to yourself or others as your source of approval or success. This is a very fearful way of living that will never produce the ideal outcome in your life. Trust God. He is your source.

TYPE 2 DIABETES

According to the Centers for Disease Control and Prevention, "more than 37 million Americans have diabetes (about 1 in 10 people), and 90 to 95 percent of them have type 2 diabetes,"[22] which has strong links to obesity. It has become a plague in our anxiety-filled and overweight nation. Type 2 diabetes is not a true disease. Do not tell your doctor I said that! That is because it is a syndrome—an anxiety and stress disorder.

A well-functioning pancreas produces insulin, the hormone that enables sugar (glucose) to move from our blood into other body cells to be used for energy. As we saw in the chapter on autoimmune disease, in type 1 diabetes, the immune system attacks the pancreas and actually destroys the pancreatic islets that produce insulin. However, in type 2 diabetes, the pancreatic islets are not diseased at all, but something invisible is stopping them from releasing the insulin properly. The cells no longer respond normally to insulin, causing the blood sugar level to rise to dangerous levels. It is a syndrome that produces an imbalance of function.

Over the years, we have found a very specific spiritual root associated with type 2 diabetes. In almost all the cases that we've seen, the person struggles with a fear of failing others. Why would we fear failing others when they are not our source? I will tell you why. Because we do not know who we are in the Father through Jesus Christ, so we look to others as our source of approval. To fail them—and thereby to not be accepted—is our greatest fear.

You must learn that you cannot depend on others accepting you. God accepts you, and that is enough. And be honest with yourself. You are not perfect, and you will fail others. But I am so thankful that God has given us the provision to repent and move on in our relationships without getting stuck in the fear of failing others. Nothing is beyond God's love and power

---

22. "Type 2 Diabetes," Centers for Disease Control and Prevention, https://www.cdc.gov/diabetes/basics/type2.html.

to heal. Psalm 103:3 tells us that He remains the God *"who forgiveth all thine iniquities; who healeth all thy diseases."*

Since type 2 diabetes is also linked to obesity, it is important for you to eat properly and to maintain a healthy weight. Remember to enjoy your favorite foods in moderation. The spiritual fruit of self-control is important as you take care of your body, which is the temple of the Holy Spirit. It is also important to take medication to manage your illness and to keep your blood sugar level under control while you work out your sanctification. Until you are set free from the spiritual root of the problem, you will still be fighting this syndrome. You will still have the fear of failing others. You may be medically managed, but you have not solved the problem until you repent of the fear, apply God's truth, and are healed.

Embrace God's Word. We have used this verse often through this journey, but the foundational Scripture for the healing of stress disorders is 1 John 4:18: *"There is no fear in love; but perfect love casteth out fear."*

All spiritually rooted disease caused by any kind of fear involves a breach in relationship at some level. It could be a breach in relationship with God; a breach in relationship with yourself, where you won't forgive yourself for your past; or a spiritual breach with someone else whom you can't forgive for hurting or abandoning you.

He that saith he is in the light, and hateth his brother, is in darkness even until now. (1 John 2:9)

How do you know there is still unforgiveness, bitterness, or hatred in your heart toward another? If you feel a zing in your spirit every time you think of that person, then you know something is wrong in your heart! Search your heart and allow the Holy Spirit to reveal which fear or breach in relationship you need to repent of. Cast down those temptations and thoughts that rise up against God's Word. Your Father loves you, and He has good things planned for your life—not rejection, fear, and disaster. Let Him transform your mind with His Word, and then rejoice in your freedom!

GASTROINTESTINAL PROBLEMS

There are a number of gastrointestinal problems caused by the spirit of fear. Much of the malfunctioning of the gastrointestinal tract is caused by not having peace in your heart regarding issues in your life.

IRRITABLE BOWEL SYNDROME

Irritable bowel syndrome (IBS) is an anxiety and stress disorder produced by a spirit of fear in which the dendrites flare in the lining of the colon, similar to how ulcers are produced in the lining of the stomach. People who have IBS likely have a compromised immune system. Bacteria grows in the colon because the immune system no longer has the firepower to defeat it. Symptoms include cramping, abdominal pain, bloating, and diarrhea or constipation. IBS is a syndrome because there is no damage to the actual large intestine or bowel tissue. Doctors consider IBS a chronic condition without a specific cause or cure.

I have observed that approximately 75 percent of those affected by IBS are female. It afflicts women who were physically or verbally abused by their fathers. Women are highly susceptible to stress disorders (and to allergies) due to a lack of love. It is the father, not the mother, who establishes the emotional well-being of his daughter first. The enemy has destroyed many homes through self-hatred in a father/husband. When a man hates himself, he will not love and care for his wife and daughter(s). If he does not believe he is loved by Father God, he will not be able to share the love of God with his family.

Remember, Satan's intent is to cause us to hate or be afraid of the word "father." Then, when we learn that God is our Father, we have a negative association based upon our experiences when we relate to Him in that role. We remain separated from our loving heavenly Father, whom we fear because of the failures of our earthly father.

I have come across many Christians, both male and female, who still feel like orphans despite knowing that Father God is their true Father according to the Bible. Just because we intellectually understand that God is not the same as our human father, we may still feel disconnected from Him. In order to overcome this serious spiritual defect, it is important to repent of any bitterness and forgive the father who abused you. As a reminder, you are not justifying sin as "okay" when you forgive. Forgiveness means that you are releasing the sin done against you and the person who sinned against you to Father God. He is the judge—not you.

When I ask an audience for a show of hands from those who never heard their father say "I love you," 80 to 90 percent of people raise their hands. Fathers are supposed to love their children well. Father God said of Jesus, *"This is my beloved Son, in whom I am well pleased." "For he received from God the Father honour and glory, when there came such a voice to him from the excellent glory, This is my beloved Son, in whom I am well pleased"* (2 Peter 1:17).

It is not sacrilegious if you say the same or similar words to your own children. I urge you to tell every one of them, from the oldest to the youngest, that you love them and that you are "well pleased" with them. Do not leave anyone out! Their health depends on it!

ULCERATIVE COLITIS

Ulcerative colitis (UC) is an inflammatory bowel disorder (IBD) that causes inflammation and ulcers (sores) in the lining of your digestive tract, particularly in the large intestines. UC is considered a stress disorder and a syndrome because even though the lining is inflamed, it is not destroyed, as it is in Crohn's disease. Symptoms include pain, abdominal cramps, and blood in the stool. Just as with the other stress disorders that we have discussed, medical science does not recognize a specific cause or cure other than some dietary and lifestyle changes. We recognize that the cure, as with the other stress disorders, is to repent of a spirit of fear and to cast down temptations enticing us to embrace the thoughts of fear for our life and fear of potential problems in our future.

MALABSORPTION, OR LEAKY GUT

Malabsorption, or leaky gut syndrome, has become a national plague. With this syndrome, the nutrients of ingested food never reach the cellular level through the bloodstream. In America, the deceptive problem behind malabsorption is that we attempt to compensate by widespread use of nutritional supplements. Unfortunately, the expensive health food and supplements also pass right on through our digestive tract without any absorption. The root behind this problem is a spirit of fear.

ACID REFLUX OR GERD

Acid reflux, or heartburn, is a common condition in which stomach acid flows back up into the esophagus. Acid reflux and gastroesophageal reflux disease (GERD) are gastrointestinal disorders brought on by a spirit of rejection. When a person is unsure whether they are accepted by others, a spirit of rejection will become a part of their life and their mindset. It will tell them they are not acceptable to God or to others—that they just do not measure up. Its armor—those evil spirits that keep rejection in our lives—include insecurity, fear of failure, fear of the future, and overall dread, increasing our fear that we have no value. As a result, we struggle to see our worth in relationships with other people.

Over sixty million Americans experience heartburn at least once a month. Some studies suggest that more than fifteen million Americans experience heartburn symptoms each day.[23] It becomes more serious when stomach acid enters the esophagus daily, causing pain, interrupting eating habits, and disturbing sleep. The condition is diagnosed as GERD when the sphincter valve that keeps the stomach acid from rising back into the esophagus is malfunctioning. Using medication and avoiding certain foods helps to manage the syndrome. Repenting of harboring a spirit of rejection and spirits of fear that reinforce its place in our lives will bring healing from GERD.

MIGRAINES

Migraines are a stress disorder with unexplained throbbing headaches, accompanied by nausea, vomiting, auras of light, fatigue, and severe mood swings. As a result of the imbalance in homeostasis that occurs, migraine sufferers have lower serotonin levels and higher histamine produced by glands in the endocrine system. Because of the increase of histamine, the blood vessels in the head expand and bump into nearby nerve tissue, causing migraine pain, which can be very intense.

---

23. NIH National Library of Medicine, "Heartburn: What you need to know," *NIH MedlinePlus Magazine*, January 21, 2020, https://magazine.medlineplus.gov/article/heartburn-what-you-need-to-know.

With migraines, there are two roots. A person is having an internal conflict about an external conflict. The external conflict is an open door for fear, which releases the histamine, and then the person feels guilt about having this conflict and how they are handling it. It may be a conflict over a relationship problem, a work situation, parenting children, or something else.

Migraines occur predominately in women. Doctors prescribe medication that will raise the serotonin levels and drop the histamine levels to control migraines. We prescribe that migraine sufferers repent of the fear and self-rejection that is tormenting them, and that they resolve their inner conflict over an external conflict by taking their peace from God and trusting Him with the relationship, the parenting issue, or whatever else the underlying conflict might be. We have seen great success in God's prescriptions.

CHRONIC INSOMNIA

Chronic insomnia is a stress disorder brought about by a spirit of fear that projects real or imagined fears, alerting the hypothalamus to go into action. Remember, the hypothalamus is like the watchdog of the endocrine system. When the hypothalamus senses stress caused by fear, it will not rest until the stress issue is resolved. The hypothalamus also controls sleep patterns, so when it is stimulated by stress, it will not allow the body to get into a restful sleep rhythm.

In order to go to sleep, you need to either arrive at a resolution or release the situation to Father God despite not knowing the outcome. It requires trusting the Lord to bring the answers for your situation in His timing, which may not be in the middle of the night! Then, the hypothalamus will stop being on continuous alert and will let you go to sleep.

I will both lay me down in peace, and sleep: for thou, LORD, only makest me dwell in safety. (Psalm 4:8)

ACNE

Acne is a skin disorder that usually affects the face, neck, back, and shoulders. Simple acne comes from the fear of man, such as peer pressure, and the fear of rejection. This level of fear and anxiety triggers increased histamine secretion behind the epidermis (skin). Histamine also increases the secretion of oil in the skin, causing acne. Those with acne, young and old, can find healing by repenting of the sins of fear of man and fear of rejection. Despite the possibility of being rejected by other people, they need to make the decision to trust Father God, believing that His acceptance is all that they need.

ASTHMA

Asthma is a stress disorder that is the product of a very specific root issue: the fear of abandonment. Over time, this spirit of fear causes a stiffening of the membrane of the air passageway. Oxygen does not get into the lungs; carbon dioxide does not get out. That causes an asthma attack. Medication will cause the air passageway to relax so that the affected person can breathe again. "A more excellent way" is to allow the Lord to deliver you from your fear. The antidote is God's promise that He will never leave you nor forsake you. Keep in mind Deuteronomy 31:6: *"Be strong and of a good courage, fear not, nor be afraid of them: for the LORD thy God, he it is that doth go with thee; he will not fail thee, nor forsake thee."*

OVEREATING

Overeating is a fear-based disorder. The spiritual roots of overeating are fear of rejection, fear of man, fear of failure, and fear of abandonment. These can be powerful forces that drive people and produce long-term anxiety and stress, both physical and mental.

Excessive eating has an addictive characteristic. All addictions are rooted in the need to be loved. A person who does not feel loved does not feel good about themselves. As a result, there is a decrease in the secretion of serotonin. Remember, serotonin is a chemical from God that makes you feel good about yourself. With a serotonin decrease, you need an upper to feel better, and you choose "comfort" food, which functions as a sort of "pacifier," a false comforter. You may gravitate toward consuming unhealthy junk food when you feel stressed. It tastes good and lulls you into a false sense of security and peace. Low serotonin also causes your metabolism to slow down, and therefore you gain weight, sometimes excessively. Since you are using comfort food to replace love, it becomes a vicious cycle.

The cure for excessive eating is to recognize spirits of fear of rejection and abandonment and repent of them. You must believe God's Word about who you are in the Father through Jesus Christ. Receive the love of God and others and quit hating yourself. The need to comfort yourself with food will diminish as you apply God's truth that you are loved in Him.

GET RID OF THE ROOT

We may ask God to heal us because of discomfort in our mind and body. However, we will not be free until we get rid of the spiritual root problem of sin. If we do not address the root issues, the disease or syndrome may come back, and we will "lose our healing" because the cause has not been uprooted. Sometimes, we gain knowledge that we refuse to live by. Humans do not like rules, but if those rules are from the Lord, they are for the benefit of us all.

Remember to guard against self-pity. Some people do not even take the time to repent because they love self-pity more than faith. Again, self-pity is the "superglue from hell" that binds you to the past. We are talking about your life. You have the Spirit of God in you, so get up and let God help you get on with it!

First Corinthians 10:13 says, "*There hath no temptation taken you but such as is common to man: but God is faithful, who will not suffer you to be tempted above that ye are able; but will with the temptation also make a way to escape, that ye may be able to bear it.*"

None of the fears that have come your way are exclusive to you. We are all tempted to embrace fear of man, fear of rejection, and other fears. We are all tempted to become anxious and stressed over the details or crises of our lives. How we handle the temptation makes all the difference. "*And ye shall know the truth, and the truth shall make you free*" (John 8:32).

Whether your healing occurs right away or takes a while in the journey, God's Word is still truth. If your healing does not occur instantly after you repent to Father God, which is what happened in Emily's testimony, then set your face like flint and determine to follow the Word of God regardless of what you feel. Draw a line in the sand and say, "No further with the lies, Satan, in Jesus's name!" "*For the Lord God will help me; therefore shall I not be confounded: therefore have I set my face like a flint, and I know that I shall not be ashamed"* (Isaiah 50:7).

YOU ARE NOT ALONE IN THE BATTLE!

The choice is yours. The Holy Spirit is your Helper. He will enable you to "walk out" of Satan's kingdom one day at a time. We don't mean to say that you are not currently following Father God, but in areas where you have allowed sin to rule your decision-making you have followed Satan's kingdom. As you repent of sin, you are choosing whom you will serve and course correcting your life. As you trust Father God with uncertain situations, you are choosing to serve Him, and you are "walking out," as we term it. With the Holy Spirit's help, you are "walking out" of the desolation of Satan's kingdom and walking into enjoying the blessings of Father God's kingdom instead.

And I will pray the Father, and he shall give you another Comforter, that he may abide with you for ever; even the Spirit of truth; whom the world cannot receive, because it seeth him not, neither knoweth him: but ye know him; for he dwelleth with you, and shall be in you.

(John 14:16–17)

You are not alone in the battle! The Holy Spirit is with you to teach you and embolden you to overcome Satan's kingdom. You ought to be a shining light of God's mercy, greatness, power, health, and sanity. You should not represent the opposite characteristics. This is vital for solving problems that seem clinical and scientific. Your spirituality impacts your health in every dimension!

WE WANT YOU TO WIN THIS BATTLE

As you know, our ministry has been active for over thirty years. However, if people are not listening to God, why would they listen to us? Our counsel is for those who desire to hear from the Word of God. If they disagree with the Bible or refuse to read it, then that is the core problem.

Many people have come to Be in Health hoping we can tell them how to receive healing despite their rebellion against the Word of God. We cannot do that. We will only give them the truth of God's Word, not some kind of psychological humanism.

Let me remind you of something. In all our years of ministry, we have been unable to help one single individual who would not take responsibility for their life. Why? Because they lacked faith according to the Word of God—biblical faith founded on God's Word, believing what He has said and acting upon it. The Bible tells us that to please God, we must have faith. *"But without faith it is impossible to please him: for he that cometh to God must believe that he is, and that he is a rewarder of them that diligently seek him"* (Hebrews 11:6).

God will not force any of us to listen to Him and agree with Him. You need to embrace the truth for yourself, and yourself alone. You must take ownership of your life in order to repent and be healed. It is time to step out in faith, trusting Father God will work with you to reform your character and nature. You must decide to repent of sin, follow the Word of God, and be an overcomer, facing fears in your life and defeating them in the name of Jesus! You can also take ownership in the victory!

We want you to win this battle! We want you to come out of the cocoon of oblivion, to come out of your place of complacency, and decide to be an overcoming believer who can defeat the enemy. As we get the victory over disease in our own lives, then we can teach others how to have victory over it, as well. We have a gift to give to humanity that even the medical world cannot give because they do not understand the spiritual problem or the spiritual solution. We understand it because the Word of God has supplied all the wisdom that we need to defeat disease. Choose to be an overcomer!

HEALED OF INVASIVE BREAST CANCER

JODY

I was diagnosed with invasive breast cancer, but the medical therapies weren't working. At the end of my chemotherapy treatments, the doctors said, "We're sorry, Jody, the mass is still large. It hasn't changed at all. You will need to have a mastectomy." I returned home and went before the Lord. God convicted me that I had unforgiveness and bitterness in my heart that I needed to deal with. The names of certain people came flooding into my mind. I needed to deal with forgiving each of them.

Each time I dealt with these things that were on my heart, the lump in my breast felt a little different. I asked the Lord, "God, is this just my imagination? What else should I be dealing with?" The issues of fear and control came to my heart. I confessed them to the Lord, and over the following days, the mass continued to decrease. When I went to the doctors to be checked one last time before the surgery, my surgeon said to me, "Jody, I can no longer recommend surgery for you. Cancer grows; it doesn't shrink. You do not need to have surgery."

Soon after, the cancer was all gone. No surgery, no chemo, no radiation. God had healed me completely of breast cancer because of the principles in His Word. I give all the glory to God! I am so very thankful! I am changed!

ELEVEN

WHAT'S NEXT?

We have exposed the spiritual roots of many diseases through the knowledge of biblical truth. Let's review a few foundational truths concerning the healing of disease.

First, spiritually rooted disease is a result of separation from God, separation from yourself, or separation from others. Therefore, all healing of spiritually rooted disease begins with reconciliation with God—receiving His love, embracing Him as your Father, and making your peace with Him. Reconciliation with yourself and with others are the next essential steps.

Second, we recognize that there are two kingdoms waging war on the inside of us: the law of sin and the law of God. Remember, even the apostle Paul expressed our need to be set free from the temptations and the roots of sin in our lives through Jesus Christ: *"For I delight in the law of God after the inward man: but I see another law in my members, warring against the law of my mind, and bringing me into captivity to the law of sin which is in my members. O wretched man that I am! who shall deliver me from the body of this death? I thank God through Jesus Christ our Lord"* (Romans 7:22–25).

Third, once we are delivered from these roots, it becomes our responsibility to renew our minds and change those old patterns of ungodly thinking. Casting down evil imaginations and filling yourself with the Word of God in your thought life is your responsibility. *"Casting down imaginations, and every high thing that exalteth itself against the knowledge of God, and bringing into captivity every thought to the obedience of Christ"* (2 Corinthians 10:5).

At Be in Health, we call this process "Walk Out". We even have a retreat we call Walk Out Workshop or WOW, because we know how important it is walking out the process of our sanctification and staying on track with the biblical truths that set us free from disease.

FOLLOW THROUGH TO DEFEAT THE ENEMY

I want to encourage you to follow through with your complete freedom from disease. Don't let the enemy discourage you. Everybody wants to be prayed for, but not everyone will follow up by defeating the lies of the enemy and embracing God's truth. Remember this Scripture: *"Ye shall know the truth, and the truth shall make you free"* (John 8:32). What I have been teaching you is designed to give you the truth and the faith to believe. This is not blind faith, but real faith based on the knowledge of a living God revealed in the Bible.

Now, I am not looking for people to become intellectually converted here. Intellectually converted people are described in Scripture: *"Ever learning, and never able to come to the knowledge of the truth"* (2 Timothy 3:7). You must cross the barrier of intellectual understanding to be led by the Holy Spirit. I didn't write this book to fill your head with a bunch of knowledge. I wrote it to break the power of the devil working in your life and to release you. Your freedom was paid for over two thousand years ago on the cross, and the power of God was released into your life so that you could live in freedom. Father God wants you to be free!

MEDITATING ON GOD'S WORD

Remember, God trains you in righteousness as you meditate, or dwell on, His Word. How often does God say to meditate on the Word? Day and night.

Blessed is the man that walketh not in the counsel of the ungodly, nor standeth in the way of sinners, nor sitteth in the seat of the scornful. But his delight is in the law of the LORD; and in his law doth he meditate day and night. (Psalm 1:1–2)

What does it mean to meditate on God's Word? The best picture I can think of is that of a cow chewing its cud. Does that sound strange? A cow doesn't just chew its food and swallow it. It chews the food to soften it, swallows it, and then regurgitates it back into its mouth to chew it again. We need to do something similar when we meditate on God's Word. We take a Scripture verse or passage and not merely read it once but rather feed on it for some time. We take in the Word, ponder it, pray about it, memorize it, and talk about it with God and with others. In that way, God's Word becomes a part of our long-term memory, a part of our personality. God uses the process of protein synthesis to build long-term memory when we dwell on His Word, but so does the enemy when we dwell on his lies.

Satan has a counterfeit for biblical meditation. During the For My Life retreat, we have a specific class dedicated to the subject of occultism, exposing occult or pagan practices not found in the Bible. As discussed earlier, it is our position that practicing "mindless meditation," as in New Age or Eastern religion, opens us up to evil spirits to torment us through the theta brain waves. When people clear their mind of all thoughts and go mindless, they are opening themselves up to an ungodly spiritual influence. It is my suspicion that this type of *theta* brainwave activity is evidence of an evil spirit speaking to a human. The reason people often feel like they are having a spiritual experience during this mindless meditation is precisely because they are, but it is *not* a good spiritual experience.

It is important to understand that when the enemy comes along, he does not give you a thought just a few times. He may give you a thought every day for 365 days a year, for years on end, because he wants to train you to have a disorder or disease. You are in his sights because you lack understanding of Satan's devices and schemes. It is our desire to continue opening your eyes to the evil devices of the enemy.

RENEWING YOUR MIND

As I have shared, Father God desires us to be free from conforming to the world by being *renewed* in our minds.

I beseech you therefore, brethren, by the mercies of God, that ye present your bodies a living sacrifice, holy, acceptable unto God, which is your reasonable service. And be not conformed to this world: but be ye trans-formed by the renewing of your mind, that ye may prove what is that good, and acceptable, and perfect, will of God. (Romans 12:1–2)

How does your mind become renewed? By being cleansed from Satan's lies and thought patterns with the washing of the water of the Word: *"That he might sanctify and cleanse it* [the church] *with the washing of water by the word"* (Ephesians 5:26).

This is why God wants us to meditate on His Word day and night, evaluating our thoughts and comparing them to how He thinks. The Word of God teaches us how to think righteously. A renewed mind is now able to confront bad thinking. This is how we become spiritual people in how we think, speak, and act. It is the journey of sanctification. Renewing our minds in God's Word allows us to build new pathways of thought. We will learn how God wants us to think and apply it to our lives.

It is our calling at Be in Health to present the truth and compel you to face your fears, your anxieties, and your sins. Father God gave us this truth to share for a very good reason. You are supposed to be changed from the ways that the world thinks and the way that it acts because that is Satan's domain. As a result, you will be delivered from the diseases that the world gets. I ask Father God to join you in your journey so that you can live in health and wholeness.

WE ARE CALLED TO BE THRIVERS!

After hearing this teaching, some people may say, "Well, this is just too much work. I would rather just take a pill and make it go away." But they will remain in captivity, waiting for some magical formula to remove the Word's requirement that we work out our own salvation: *"Wherefore, my beloved, as ye have always obeyed, not as in my presence only, but now much more in my absence, work out your own salvation with fear and trembling"* (Philippians 2:12). I have to work out my own salvation every day. I have to make up my mind about which law I will follow. On any given day, I have to cast out thoughts and feelings that are not of God. Don't you?

One of my greatest griefs is that while God has given our Be in Health team a measure of truth to give to others that they might be healed from disease, some people, when they hear the truth, become offended at the suggestion that any of their physical infirmities could be because of a failure to think, speak, or act the way God says to. Or, they hear the message and appear to embrace it, but then just don't follow through with claiming their identities and renewing their mind in God's truth. I pray that you will follow through, then God will come and heal you.

You were not called to be one of God's own just to be a survivor—you were called to be a *thriver*. The world is full of survivors. You should be a thriver! While the world might be struggling in disease and hopelessness, you should be a happy, well balanced, and enthusiastic son or daughter of God. You should be excited to be here on this planet.

BEING CHANGED INTO GOD'S IMAGE

Never forget that you are being changed into God's image as you follow His Word. *"But we all, with open face beholding as in a glass the glory of the Lord, are changed into the same image from glory to glory, even as by the Spirit of the Lord"* (2 Corinthians 3:18). Don't let anyone steal the truths that you have learned here. People with unbelief will try to debate you, discourage you, and drag you down to their image. You are not being formed into the image of any other person. You're being transformed into the image of God! As you are being changed into His image, you can expect God to heal you from the diseases of the enemy because God honors His Word and His image. He honors who He is in you, not at the head level, but at the heart level.

Through Jesus Christ, the Father is recapturing and recovering what He lost in the tragedy of the garden of Eden—His image in mankind. That is the power of the cross. You are a product of that recovery and restoration. You are being called out of darkness and being changed into His marvelous light. *"But ye are a chosen generation, a royal priesthood, an holy nation, a peculiar people; that ye should shew forth the praises of him who hath called you out of darkness into his marvellous light"* (1 Peter 2:9). But you cannot be *transformed* unless you are *reformed* by the Word, because *"faith cometh by hearing, and hearing by the Word of God"* (Romans 10:17).

GOD WANTS TO MAKE YOU FREE

Even though it may feel uncomfortable to confront certain issues brought up in this teaching, I implore you to address them. God loves you, and you're not reading this book just because you feel like it. You are reading this because the Spirit of God wants to set you and your loved ones free from disease. When I became a believer, there were words burning inside of me. I was not called to be an evangelist, but I was called to use those words to bring healing, deliverance, and hope to God's people.

Do not let anyone tell you that you're not the apple of God's eye. (See Deuteronomy 32:10.) Do not let anybody ever tell you that you are not engraved in the palm of His hands. (See Isaiah 49:16.) Do not let anyone ever tell you that your name is not written down in the Book of Life (see, for example, Revelation 3:5), or that you are not a son or daughter of the Father (see, for example, Galatians 4:6-7). Don't let anyone interfere with who you are. You are not an accident; you were a planned event by God. Before you were ever conceived, God knew you; before your body parts began to form, He said, "You are mine."

Before I formed thee in the belly I knew thee; and before thou camest forth out of the womb I sanctified thee. (Jeremiah 1:5)

But now thus saith the LORD that created thee, O Jacob, and he that formed thee, O Israel, Fear not: for I have redeemed thee, I have called thee by thy name; thou art mine. (Isaiah 43:1)

Are you struggling in any of these areas of God's love for you? Are you afraid that you are not up to the task of changing your thought patterns? Breathe in and breathe out. Let God renew you. Don't embrace the spirit of death. God has created you with a purpose and a plan, and He has created you to live. It is the enemy who has a plan for you to die.

Relax. You are not your disease. You are not the problem; the devil is. Stop listening to him. Choose life; don't choose death. Be kind to yourself. Live in this dispensation of grace and mercy. Choose life and not death.

My prayer for you: "Father, I come to You in the name of Jesus. I want to thank You for this precious person who has taken the time to read this book. I know from Psalm 139 in Your Word that they are fearfully and wonderfully made, and Your hand is upon each and every one of them. I know that I have given them many things to think about from Your Word. I ask You to release Your Holy Spirit to bring understanding and conviction, so that they made be changed from the inside out, and that their diseases would vanish.

"Father, we are just people, men and women from many different backgrounds. We have listened to lies we didn't know were lies; we have pursued things we thought were right but are leading to our destruction. Please show us the good way where there is rest for our souls. Teach us to grow up in this thing called life and mature as sons and daughters of God. Let this be, Father, so that we may be whole in spirit, soul, and body, and that the generations after us would also be whole and a light to the world of Your glory, goodness, and love toward us. Thank You so much for Your mercy, Sir, and continue to teach us by Your grace. In Jesus's name I pray. Amen."

WHAT BE IN HEALTH OFFERS

Now that we've exposed the spiritual roots of diseases, you may be interested in these other resources that Be in Health˚ has to offer:

FOR MY LIFE®

For My Life is a one-week retreat hosted by Be in Health at our campus in Thomaston, Georgia. It is designed to help people who are seeking healing and restoration of their physical, emotional, and spiritual health. We believe that most diseases result from separation in relationship from God, ourselves, and others. This retreat will help you to identify and deal with the root issues that may be keeping you from being in health.

The For My Life Retreat consists of intensive teachings, group ministry sessions, time to interact with the teachers and ask questions, and a time for personal prayer for healing at the end of the week. Be in Health endeavors to make For My Life a safe place for you to find hope and healing for your life.

WALK OUT® WORKSHOP (WOW)

After For My Life, the next step is the Walk Out Workshop (WOW). The term "walk out" refers to the journey of walking out of the old life of disease and hopelessness and entering into a new life of health and wholeness. During this one-week workshop, our team and attendees roll up their sleeves and begin to get really interactive with the principles from For My Life.

We address topics such as how to not go into guilt when we fall short, becoming established in our identity, overcoming temptation, how to forgive when you've been hurt, and learning to walk in the Father's love. Break-out groups, lots of Q & A, and continued healing of your spirit, soul, and body are all part of this amazing week.

FOR MY LIFE EXPANDED (4MLX)

The For My Life eXpanded Retreat is our brand-new, next in series, five-day retreat, which will take you even deeper into the Be in Health teachings. Develop a profound understanding of the specific spiritual roots of major disease classes and discover powerful insights into healing and recovery in God. This retreat will set you on the next level of your Overcomers' Journey. There are also corporate times of ministry through-out the week.

FOR MY LIFE KIDS AND FOR MY LIFE YOUTH

Every year in June and July, we offer For My Life for the whole family; that is the For My Life Adult, For My Life Youth (ages 13–17), and For My Life Kids (ages 6–12) Retreats all in the same week! This is an opportunity for the whole family to be transformed and healed from the inside out.

We hear so many people say, "If only I had known this when I was younger, I would have been saved from so much torment and heartache!" We've listened and developed these specialized retreats to continue our mission of establishing generations of overcomers. In the For My Life family week, everybody in the family can benefit and be on the same page spiritually. We take the same information that is presented in the adult For My Life Retreat but reformat it to be relevant and engaging for each audience.

WOW KIDS

After the For My Life family weeks, we have the WOW family weeks. This is an opportunity for the whole family to come and learn how to be overcomers together. The WOW Kids class (ages 6–12) will equip your children with the skills that they need to be overcomers. With a fun, engaging format, games, activities, and special "tools for freedom," your kids are sure to have a blast, make lasting memories, make new friends, and come out with valuable resources that will help them on their Overcomers' Journey throughout their lives.

 To learn more about the Be in Health Retreats, visit: www.beinhealth.com/for-my-life

THE OVERCOMERS' COMMUNITY®

The journey of being an overcomer can be challenging, and we don't want you to have to do it alone. That is why we've developed the Overcomers' Community. This is a membership-based online forum dedicated to being a safe place for you to connect with the Be in Health Team as well as with other overcomers. You can ask questions, get support and encouragement, share testimonies, find specific spiritual roots of diseases, have access to a wide selection of complete teachings, and more! We look forward to joining you and assisting you in your Overcomer's Journey. With God's help, we can do this together!

 To learn more about the Overcomers' Community, visit www.beinhealth.com/overcomers-community.

BE IN HEALTH CONFERENCES NEAR YOU

Our Be in Health Team travels too! We bring one- to three-day conferences to locations all over the world. If you want to find out more about these conferences and when one might be held in your area, or if you are interested in helping us bring a conference to your area, go to **www.beinhealth.com.**

SPIRITUAL LIFELINE®

Spiritual Lifeline is a ministry of love and personal assistance from the Be in Health team; it is our most individualized form of ministry to you. Our Father promises to deliver us from the enemy as we apply His Word.

Together, we'll look at God's plan for your situation and His promises that will sustain you. Private ministry and prayer sessions are provided over the phone or through an online voice- or video-calling platform.

Spiritual Lifeline is not a starting place at Be in Health. It is designed to come alongside and assist those who have previously attended our For My Life Retreat or have read and are applying the principles of Dr. Wright's books *A More Excellent Way* and *Exposing the Spiritual Roots of Disease*.

 To learn more about Spiritual Lifeline, visit www.beinhealth.com/phone-ministry.

HEALTH RESOURCES

You can find all the information that we offer on specific disease and mental health topics. Under each topic, all the relevant Be in Health teachings, conferences, blogs, YouTube videos, healing testimonies, and related resources are categorized so you can find everything you need in one place. We continue to add new content, so keep checking back for more of the information you are looking for!

 Discover our Health Resources at www.beinhealth.com/healing-resources.

PNEUMAPSYCHOSOMATOLOGY® (PPS).

PneumaPsychoSomatology®: Pneuma (spirit) – Pyscho (soul) – Soma (body) – tology (the study of)

After decades of working with people and disease, Dr. Henry W. Wright developed a new type of scientific study called PneumaPsychoSomatology, or PPS. PPS is just a word for the study of the connection between the spirit, soul, and body.

The Bible is clear about the enemy's kingdom and how spirits, such as fear, affect people on the earth. There are also many Scriptures that indicate how our disobedience to God and agreement with these spirits can cause disease in our bodies. *"Men's hearts failing them for fear, and for looking after those things which are coming on the earth: for the powers of heaven shall be shaken"* (Luke 21:26).

BE IN HEALTH BOOKSTORE

If you enjoyed this book, you will love our other books and teaching resources in the Be in Health Bookstore. You will find an extensive selection of materials by Dr. Henry W. Wright, Pastor Donna Wright, and other

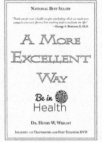

leadership team members. Topics range from the possible spiritual roots of diseases to how to overcome specific spiritual issues to teachings on sound biblical doctrine.

A More Excellent Way

Dr. Henry W. Wright's book *A More Excellent Way* is our number one resource, selling over 300,000 copies worldwide. It is an excellent, comprehensive introduction to the root causes behind diseases and how to overcome them in your life. Included in the back of the book are 150 healing

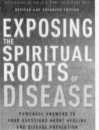

testimonies and a free teaching DVD.

Exposing the Spiritual Roots of Disease

In *Exposing the Spiritual Roots of Disease*, Dr. Wright presents a thoroughly biblical and compelling case for healing. If you think you've read all you need to know about healing, it's time to take another look! Dr. Wright clearly shows that disease is not a random occurrence and that science and medicine have their place in dealing with illness but can only offer disease management. What if the answers to true healing have been in the Bible all along?

Find these books and more in the Be in Health Bookstore: resources.beinhealth.com.

BE IN HEALTH BLOG

The Be in Health Blog offers biblical insights in a selection of articles about spiritual principles, overcoming, roots to diseases, and more. In addition, there are inspiring testimonies that are sure to encourage you in your own Overcomers' Journey.

 Find our blog at www.beinhealth.com/blog.

HOPE OF THE GENERATIONS CHURCH

Be in Health is a ministry of Hope of the Generations Church (HGC), a local body of believers located in Thomaston, Georgia. HGC is a non-denominational church and follows the model of the first-century church that was set in place by the apostles. We believe that every church, regardless of its background or diversity, should witness the same things recorded in the Bible: signs, wonders, healings, and miracles. These are life-altering tools of God to establish the authenticity of His Word.

Join us Sunday mornings at 10:00 a.m. EST or Friday nights at 7:00 p.m. EST.

We also stream our church services on our YouTube channel: www.youtube.com/beinhealth.

A.C.T.S. GLOBAL;
ASSOCIATION OF CHURCHES TEACHING AND SERVING®

Have you considered that God may be calling you to start, pastor, and establish a local church or gathering? Have the teachings of Be in Health opened your eyes, and now you want to tell others? Do you love people and want to see God's best for their lives?

Do you have a desire to guard the purity of the Bible and share that with others? Do you already, or do you desire to, gather people together to grow, heal, and fellowship together? Do people come to you for help and direction for their lives? Are you ready to be a pastor but are held back by a lack of resources and training?

If you answered yes to one or more of these questions, A.C.T.S. Global is here to help you take the next step.

 To learn more about A.C.T.S. Global, visit www.actsglobal.com.

BE IN HEALTH E-MAIL LIST

Do you want to stay connected with Be in Health and receive updates, messages from our pastors, news, events, and blog posts directly in your inbox?

 Sign up for Be in Health's mailing list at www.beinhealth.com.

SOCIAL MEDIA

You can also follow us on your favorite social-media platforms!

Facebook: @beinhealth

Instagram: beinhealth

Twitter: @BeinHealth

YouTube: www.youtube.com/beinhealth

Pinterest: bnhealth

ABOUT THE AUTHOR

Dr. Henry Wright believed that many human problems, particularly as they relate to health, are fundamentally spiritual with resulting psychological and biological manifestations. Because of his extensive research and insights into both the medical and spiritual aspects of disease, he developed a unique and fresh perspective on ministering to the sick. Through over thirty years of application, ministry, and personal experience, Dr. Wright discovered that many diseases have an often-overlooked spiritual root that must be identified and dealt with from a biblical perspective in order for true healing to occur. He successfully applied these principles in teaching and ministering to others, with astounding results, as God healed many people from their diseases, many of which were considered incurable.

Dr. Wright grew up knowing that God heals disease. Two months after his birth, his mother was dying of fibrosarcoma cancer with an aggressive tumor that had wrapped itself around her jugular vein. At church one Sunday, she repented of bitterness and cried out to God. Instantly, the tumor disappeared. One week later, her doctor was amazed to find no evidence of cancer in her body. No medical treatment had been administered. Consequentially, her healing broke a genetic pattern in her generations; her own mother had died of cancer soon after giving birth to her. She went on to live thirty-three more years! Her prayer was that her son would someday serve God too. Though she didn't see the fruit of that prayer in her lifetime, God was faithful to place a calling on Dr. Wright's life. Her healing set a standard within him against the enemy and against disease.

Dr. Wright held a doctorate in Christian Therapeutic Counseling from Chesapeake Bible College in Ridgeley, Maryland. He was the president and founder of Be in Health Global® and the senior pastor of Hope of the Generations Church (HGC) in Thomaston, Georgia. Henry and his wife, Donna, faithfully taught and ministered to those who God sent to them. They also traveled all over the world, teaching in conferences and ministering about healing in Jesus's name. Over time, they established the impactful For My Life Retreat in Thomaston, as well as other retreats. These retreats have brought tens of thousands of people to restoration and healing in God as they discovered the spiritual roots of disease and applied scriptural truths to their whole lives—spirit, soul, and body.

Dr. Wright's first book, *A More Excellent Way* is a best-seller in the Christian market, has been translated into seven languages, and has sold hundreds of thousands of copies worldwide. It has helped thousands of people recover from the devastation of disease and find healing in God's plan. His book *Exposing the Spiritual Roots of Disease* also provides biblical truths to those seeking answers for disease.

Dr. Henry Wright passed away on November 18, 2019. Because of his passion for the Be in Health ministry to accomplish the Father's will for generations to come, Dr. Wright, his ministry team, and the board of directors had already established plans for the future. Dr. Wright's vision and ministry continue under the leadership of Hope of the Generations' Senior Pastors Scott and Sarah Harper, son-in-law and daughter of the Wrights. Pastor Scott also serves as the CEO of Be in Health. Pastor Donna Wright, Dr. Henry's wife and co-founder of HGC and Be in Health, is actively involved with both the church and the ministry. Along with the other pastors and elders of HGC, she continues to invest her life into carrying forth the vision of Dr. Wright.

Today, thousands of people are still welcomed to the Be in Health campus each year and to conferences around the country as Dr. Wright's legacy continues to bring healing and restoration to the people who God sends to them.